Caring

Making a Difference One Story at a Time

Collected and Compiled by
Terry L. Bream
Joyce A. Johnson

Editor
Karen B. Casady

Inspired by
Linda Fahey

Editorial Board
Susan Al-Sabih, Ilene Gelbaum, Kris Hillary,
Rosanne Padovich and Teri Pitman

With the assistance of
Kathy Christmas, Denise Duncan and Patty Hayden

KAISER PERMANENTE®
Southern California

Anne
Gold Fisher
CNO
851-7742

Project Management and Coordination: Communications Plus
Editor: Karen B. Casady
Cover, Interior Book Design and Production: Robin Weisz/Graphic Design and The Oak Company

Dedicated to

the staff and physicians of Kaiser Permanente

and to the members they serve

with pride and devotion

The quilt on the cover of "Caring: Making a Difference One Story at a Time"
is a patchwork quilt. Each patch is different and that's the beauty of it.
So, just as the quilt comes together with a multitude of color and patterns
so it is with this book; a coming together of stories reflecting the many
of us who work at Kaiser Permanente and our shared wisdom, strength,
knowledge and fortitude.

Table of Contents

Foreword

This book, *Caring: Making a Difference One Story at a Time*, is about the people of Kaiser Permanente. It represents an extraordinary effort from those providers who, each day, define and deliver care and compassion at the bedside. It reinforces our philosophy: "Our cause is health. Our passion is service. We're here to make lives better." The stories in this book illustrate the values of our organization and convey how they surface within patient care experiences.

Today the delivery of health care is far too complex for any one profession to do alone. Everything plays out at the bedside but it plays out through a superbly blended lineup of people. It takes an integrated team to pull together good health care. This book is a fine example of that collaboration, its stories representing virtually all settings where we provide care.

The health of our organization depends on the loyalty and perceptions of our patients and their decision to choose Kaiser Permanente. An organization is only as good as the people who make it up. The stories in this book are exquisite examples of our commitment to excellence.

As physicians, we realize the value of partnership and the role it plays in creating the reputation of our organization. We are delighted with the individuals who took the time and made the effort to share their stories and experiences. Often we find ourselves too busy to step back and recognize the great work that goes on at

Kaiser Permanente. *Caring: Making a Difference One Story at a Time* goes to that point and beyond. We are humbled by the examples in this book and proud to be colleagues of the writers and the team who created it.

Benjamin K. Chu, MD, MPH
President
Southern California Region
Kaiser Foundation Health Plan, Inc.
and Hospitals

Jeffrey A. Weisz, MD
Executive Medical Director
Southern California Permanente Medical
Group

"Cure sometimes, treat often, comfort always."
Hippocrates

Introduction

"It takes a thousand voices to tell a single story."
Native American saying

We think they had it right and we have it right. Because, in publishing this book, we have taken the voices of Kaiser Permanente, joined them together and told our single most important story. We have gathered the experiences of many and are now telling the world about who we are, what we do and how we care. We are sharing our wisdom, strength, knowledge and fortitude.

Caring: Making a Difference One Story at a Time began as a purposeful attempt to create a legacy and to document our history and heritage. We asked people to "Share a special moment. Savor your memories. Leave a legacy. Tell us your story." Our providers responded in kind.

We thought we were setting our sights high when we decided on a goal of 60 stories as a measure of success. The enthusiastic response showed us that people were willing to take the risk to write about and submit an experience that happened to them.

We now have a collection of 100 wonderful stories and poems. We drew out and put down on paper personal accounts of wisdom, passion, humor and heroism. There are quiet stories and boisterous stories; there are miracle stories and funny stories. We have tearful stories about death and dying balanced with stories about wondrous births. We span the continuum of life.

We have created a sacred bundle in the spirit of ancestral tradition where stories were gathered and told, passing along history and culture. We are writing down the sacred bundle of stories about those of us who provide care. We are drawing out and putting down on paper the lore and the legends that Kaiser Permanente providers live every day.

Each story is a gift, an insight into another human being, a written, shared and collegial experience. This book has connected us to each other in new ways. Think of what we have gained. Telling our stories has empowered us in terms of our roles in health care. We have learned the importance of who we are and of how we make a difference.

One of the goals of this book project was to get in touch with why we became nurses and care providers in the first place. We have discovered that self-knowledge can uplift us wherever we find ourselves. These are our stories, our demonstrated impact and our legacy.

Caring: Making a Difference One Story at a Time was a deliberate, purposeful, reflective effort to collect the stories we knew were out there and publish them. Bravo and kudos to all! We did it!

Terry Bream, RN, MN
Administrator
Ambulatory Clinical Services
Southern California Permanente
Medical Group

Linda Fahey, RN, NP, MSN
Regional Manager
Quality and Patient Safety
Patient Care Services
Kaiser Permanente Southern California

Acknowledgements

Caring: Making a Difference One Story at a Time began with the vision of two people, Linda Fahey and me. In 2007, Linda passionately brought the work of Quint Studer to my attention. She had attended a Studer Group conference and brought back a book called *What's Right in Health Care: 365 Stories of Purpose, Worthwhile Work and Making a Difference.*

From that moment, a dream grew. Whereas Quint Studer reinforced my passion for the value of storytelling, Linda told me with great certainty and promise that we too had those stories and that they needed sharing. She had the knowledge and forethought to see the great merit of publishing a collection of Kaiser Permanente stories.

Linda and I have a wonderful relationship and share a mutual commitment to our nursing profession, to our colleagues and ultimately to our members. Based on that dedication, we both felt an intense need to manifest this project. I am indebted to Linda, because without her inspiration, this book would not have come to fruition.

This project officially began in late 2007. This is not a venture that one does alone, or even with one or two other people. To that end, I put together what has become a cohesive, hard-working team. Our numbers ebbed and flowed, depending on what needed doing, but there always remained a core group of dedicated people from close at hand to the far reaches of the Kaiser Permanente Southern California

Region. They represent many types of practice and came from the ambulatory side as well as the hospital and health plan side of our organization.

Teri Pitman's buoyant enthusiasm carried us through many a moment. Rosanne Padovich consistently put one foot in front of the other, shouldering many a boring burden and seeing them through to the end. Ilene Gelbaum edited and edited and edited. And every once in awhile, we'd get these phenomenally creative cards from Ilene with all of our smiling faces riding happily on the page. I have mine framed on my desk.

Sue Al-Sabih became our legal authority and voice of reason, keeping us anchored during our occasionally unreasonable flights of fancy. Kris Hillary edited, wisely commented and brought with her many stories from her home health colleagues.

Others who jumped in to help, particularly when we were reading and scoring story after story, were Patty Hayden, Denise Duncan and Kathy Christmas. Without their assistance, we would not have gotten through the many, many stories that we received.

Joyce Johnson and Karen Casady were the lynchpins of this adventure. Karen managed and copyedited the entire project, from start to finish. To put it bluntly, the book would not have happened without her. But, she could not have done her work without Joyce, her Kaiser Permanente partner. These two worked in concert with each other, in perfect harmony, to carry the metaphor a bit further. They met, tweaked, rolled up their sleeves and melded their brains together on nearly every issue that arose over the long course of putting this book together. They were then, and remain now, two very remarkable people.

There are so many others. Judy Husted, representing the hospital and health plan of Kaiser Permanente, helped with funding the project. My boss, Tom Williamson, encouraged me and gave me the leeway to produce this book. My assistant, Teresa Sides, kept me organized and helped tremendously with the nitty-gritty of ISBN numbers and the like.

Outside of Kaiser Permanente, there is Robin Weisz, who patiently worked with us on the design of this book and Lesley Zanich who painstakingly set the type. Tim Casady became an invaluable resource to my editor who had numerous clinical questions to ask her nurse husband. Finally, Dr. Robert L. Patten, Lynette S. Autrey Professor in Humanities, Department of English, Rice University advised on various editorial matters.

Finally, thank you to everyone who wrote and submitted a story, published or not. It takes courage to set pen to paper and then send it out. We gathered quite an array of written pieces from people all over the region, with various credentials and in different practice roles. Without you and your efforts, we would have no book.

There remains one more group to thank—our members and patients. In a very real way, we owe them a debt of gratitude. They are the people for whom we care. They allow us to be of service and to pursue our chosen professions in health care. Our stories stem from our interactions with them. We have all grown from the experience of creating this book.

Thank you…thank you…thank you!

Terry Bream, RN, MN
Administrator
Ambulatory Clinical Services
Southern California Permanente Medical Group

"Storytelling is the most powerful way to put ideas into the world today."
Robert McKee

A Baby Needs His Mother and a Mother Needs Her Baby

The patient was in the ICU, unconscious and on a ventilator following a seizure and brain herniation from pregnancy-induced hypertension. Her baby was in the newborn nursery.

I had just returned from a three-day, skin-to-skin bonding program. I brought her baby up to the ICU, unwrapped him and removed his T-shirt. I lowered the patient's hospital gown and placed the baby skin-to-skin on her chest. Before I placed the baby on her chest, I called her by name and told her that her son was here. It was a good chance to put into practice what I had just learned.

The baby spent several minutes lying cheek to chest. Several times, he attempted to make eye contact with his mother, adjusting his position and trying to see her. But, the ventilator tube always obstructed his view.

After about 30 minutes, the baby had positioned himself on his mother's chest so that he was able to latch onto her breast and breastfeed successfully. As he suckled, his left hand was on the ventilator tube pushing it ever so slightly to remove it from his line of sight to his mother's face. He gazed up at her lovingly.

Several days later, the mother regained consciousness and was extubated. As I entered her room, I introduced myself. She stopped me mid sentence.

"I know who you are," she said. "You are the one who brought my baby to me. Until I felt him on my chest, I was unclear about where I was or what had happened. When I heard you say my baby was here and I felt him against my skin, I began to understand my situation. When I felt him latch onto my breast, I knew I had to fight to stay alive because my baby needs his mother."

The hospital discharged mom and baby and both are doing well. I knew the physical instinct between mothers and their babies is broad and powerful. But this particular interaction influenced my care. In this case, would the mother have survived without the sense that her baby was there? I learned firsthand the importance of keeping families together even under dire circumstances. It's good for the babies and it's good for the moms.

Kathleen Long, RN, CNS
Perinatal Services, Orange County

"A mother is a person who seeing there are only four pieces of pie for five people, promptly announces she never did care for pie."
Tenneva Jordan

Upside Down

In a very old hospital sat a little boy who'd had many surgeries and would have many more before he healed. He was scared and lonely and knew from past surgeries that he would hurt after the operation was over.

I was new to the hospital and new to anesthesia, having just graduated the year before. My heart went out to this little boy who did not want an IV started but his airway and injuries were such that an IV was necessary. I tried to talk him into an IV but he was wise to all my pleadings and unequivocally said "NO!"

"If I stand on my head, will you let me start an IV?" I said without missing a beat.

"Sure, if you stand on your head," he said, certain it would never happen, being the experienced skeptic that he was.

Well, I stood on my head. For a moment, he was silent and then he laughed. He did not even move while I started the IV.

I didn't know that my new boss was standing outside the door. "What will you do next time?" she said when she saw me. We laughed and from then on, the little boy was always mine when he came for his surgeries and he always let me start the IV.

Shelly Lethiot, CRNA, EdD
Assistant Director, Kaiser Permanente School of Anesthesia, Pasadena

"Miracles come in moments. Be ready and willing."
Wayne Dyer

One Exceptional
Night Shift

I was driving back home on the Ortega Highway with my sister talking about our visit with our dad. As we chatted, I looked to the opposite lane, saw a van skid slowly sideways and go off the side of the mountain. It was like a slow motion movie scene but really happened in seconds. Both my sister and I said at the same time, "Oh my God!"

It was dusk and there was a light rain. I pulled over quickly and we looked down a very steep cliff. All we could see was dust and smoke.

"Are you okay?" I yelled.

There was no response. I kept calling and after the third try, I heard a man faintly and desperately say, "I am okay but my wife is hurt. We need help!"

"We are going to help," I called back. "We're not going to leave you."

We were the only witnesses to this accident. We could not use our cell phones because there was no reception so I started flagging down cars. I asked the first person to go to a stationary phone and call 911. The next couple who pulled over agreed to help me climb down to the accident scene. The man's name was Mike. My sister was urging us to wait for help but I knew we had to act quickly.

I grabbed a first aid kit and a blanket from the back of my car. Mike and I sat at the top of the embankment looking down at a steep 200-foot cliff and decided we could probably slide down. My adrenalin gave me the courage to go for it. Mike sat in front of me and we scooted down the cliff together but we started slipping and losing control. The van had loosened the soil and pulled away all the shrubs. There was nothing to grab.

It was obvious our plan wasn't working so we pushed ourselves back up to the top. Then Mike remembered he had a rope. We tied the rope to the back of his truck and used it to slide down together. We had just enough rope to make it to the bottom of the cliff.

The man was standing there stunned. He was not badly injured. He had many abrasions and was very anxious.

"You need to get my wife out of the van now," he said to us. The van was not stable. It was teetering on its side and it was in a creek.

Mike went to the van to help the wife. Her name was Jeanne. She was lying face down with her arms extended above her head. The exploding air bag had rocketed her to the back of the van and she had caught herself with both arms.

The van was rocking back and forth and I was concerned about fire. We needed to get Jeanne out quickly in spite of any injuries. As Mike slid her along the seat using her pants, she screamed in pain. She was able to get into a sitting position and then walk with her arms supported in front of her. We escorted her to a safer area away from the van and sat her down next to her husband.

Her injuries were definitely more serious. She had a very edematous left eye and possibly fractured arms. She also had abrasions and bruises. To my relief it appeared no one had life-threatening injuries. That in itself was a miracle. I used my supplies from the first aid kit and wrapped Jeanne with the foil blanket, which secured and supported her arms as she held them close to her body, and kept her warm.

We lit the candles from the kit because it had gotten darker and colder. While waiting for the paramedics, I monitored Jeanne. Her husband told me he'd lost control of the van on some loose gravel and could not regain his steering. The van had rolled over at least three times before hitting the cliff bottom. Things could have been much worse.

We heard the rescue team arrive. Jeanne's pain level was worse. It was now very dark, still drizzling and the crickets had joined our conversation. Finally, after what seemed an eternity, the paramedics got to us, equipped with a hoist and all their fancy gear.

"What took so long?" I asked. They told me they needed to decide whether to use a helicopter or the hoist. "Besides, it looks like you have things in control," one of them said.

"Where is the champagne?" said another. Everyone chuckled because it did look romantic, lit candles, the patients bundled in blankets and stable for the moment, the sound of crickets and a big spotlight shining on the night's scenery. The paramedics did their assessments and took Jeanne up the cliff in a basket gurney using the hoist. Her husband followed and I was last.

When I reached the top, I was so surprised. Coming from dark, quiet and composed and going to bright, hectic and hurried, it was like being in a different place. Cars were backed up for miles on the two-lane highway. There were two fire engines, two paramedic trucks, police cars and tow trucks, and police directing traffic and trying to clear the congestion. I stood there in awe!

My patient Jeanne was in the paramedic truck about to be taken to the hospital when her husband came over, shook my hand and said, "Thank you for all you did and for staying with us."

"Glad I could help," I said and gave him a hug.

That night was a first-time experience for me. I had to use my critical thinking skills in an emergency away from the hospital or clinic setting, without a doctor or any other medical people. I learned the value of a first aid kit and that emotional support can be as effective as first aid nursing skills. My patients were reassured when they needed it most. I listened and did what they asked which created a calming effect. I directed care well and the outcome was good.

I found out the extent of Jeanne's injuries through the paramedics and they let her know I was sending good wishes. Jeanne wrote such a nice thank-you note when she had recovered from her surgeries. She fractured both shoulders. The left needed an artificial shoulder replacement and the right shoulder needed plates and six screws.

In her note, she called me her "guardian angel" and said, "I will never be able to put into words the deep appreciation for your concerns and actions that evening. You gave unselfishly of yourself in an effort to help me and my husband."

I chose nursing as my career when I graduated early from high school. Over many years, I have cared for patients in numerous settings and I've worked every shift, my least favorite being the night shift. However, this one-time extraordinary nursing experience, during this particular "night shift" boosted my confidence and motivated me to be a better nurse.

Those heartfelt words of appreciation that my patient shared have inspired and acknowledged that nursing is the right fit for me. When all was said and done, I told myself, "You did well."

P.S. Mike had climbed back up the rope after he got Jeanne out of the van. I think he reported to the rescue team and left before the traffic backed up. I wish I could have thanked him for his heroic efforts.

Kathy Begin, RN
Team Leader, Family Medicine, Orange County

*"Satisfaction in your work is one of the
fruits of a wise choice."*
Eugenia Kennedy Spalding

My Gift to Our Members

Mine is not so much a story of any one event. It is more of a journey with Kaiser Permanente that has helped me to grow and has helped to shape who I am today. I was born at Kaiser Permanente Fontana in 1970 and have been a lifelong member and patient. I have seen and been through many changes with our organization.

I first became employed with Kaiser Permanente in 1992, starting in the Outpatient Records Department. Since July 2000, I have worked for the Department of Psychiatry. I am now at the Psychiatry Appointment Services Department at Palm Court in Fontana as a Psychiatry Social Clerk, scheduling appointments for our members in need.

At times, it can be trying and difficult work. However, I have found that my attitude has everything to do with my approach. When that part of me is in order, I find that my job becomes very rewarding. I have learned so much from what I do and from working with my colleagues. But, it is our patients who have been particularly good teachers.

I have acquired patience and the ability to pause and step back inwardly when faced with a difficult member on the phone. I have gained a deeper level of compassion, learning to listen with not just my ears, but with my heart. When people are suffering, it often takes a great deal of courage for them to reach out and make that call to us.

Most importantly, I know that each day I have an opportunity to make a difference in the lives of our patients. A kind word can go a long way, and even a simple acknowledgement of the other person's feelings can help them to feel validated and reassured.

You may be thinking, "All this, from an appointment clerk?"

My response is, "Why not?"

I enjoy offering my simple, human skills. I am an important part of the whole organization, and I am passionate about my work. I fill a niche and I am fulfilled by what I do every day. Our patients inspire me.

When a person shares the news that they are doing and feeling better, I am genuinely happy for them in their success. I treat each member as though he or she is the only person in the world that matters right then and there, if only for a few minutes.

Mine is the voice that soothes and comforts; this knowledge is empowering and wonderful to use every day. I give the precious gift of being heard to each and every patient who calls. And, if I am lucky, I receive a gift in return, a heartfelt, "Thank you! I feel so much better after just talking to you!"

Anna Marciano

Psychiatry Social Clerk, Department of Psychiatry, Fontana

"We must not, in trying to think about how we can make a big difference, ignore the small daily differences we can make which, over time, add up to big differences that we often cannot foresee."

Marian Wright Edelman

Nursing...An Elusive Passion

I sat in the reception area of Miss McLennan's office feeling very small and stressed, wondering if it was such a good idea to be there. I bowed my head as I begged God for strength, seeing two white legs inside a pair of spotless clinic nursing shoes standing directly in front of me.

"Miss Baba, come with me," the owner of the legs said. I followed her into the office. It occurred to me that her dress could, at the end of her day, stand on its own strength.

"How may I help you, Miss Baba?" said Miss McLennan.

"I wanted to speak with you about my rejection letter," I said.

After several rounds of "we're committed...we've evaluated...and we've concluded," Miss McLennan finally said, "You aren't, in our opinion, nursing material."

I cleared my throat and asked, "May I speak to the admittance committee?"

Silence. I am not sure how long I held my breath, but when she said yes, and I finally exhaled, I felt faint.

One week later, the same receptionist led me through closed doors into a room filled with identically dressed nurses, each with her own hat, uniform and amazingly spotless, white clinic nursing shoes.

The inquiry began. One person, sitting to my right, Miss Nelson, seemed to ask the most questions. She was the only one not smiling. At the end of their interview, they asked, "Miss Baba, do you have any questions for us?"

I did have a question, and in that split second I decided to risk all by asking it.

"Recently, the National League for Nursing questioned you regarding the 50 percent of the freshman class who flunk out of nursing school each year," I said.

I stopped for a moment but I had gone too far to quit, so I moved onto my question.

"If the 50 percent of those who fail were accepted by you as students who were capable of graduating, yet did not, then what about those students who you reject?" I asked. "Is it possible that some of them might be able to make it through nursing school, yet never have the chance to demonstrate that they can?"

Silence. From far away, I heard them dismiss me. Slowly I rose and crept out of the room, out to my car, and back to my job at Franklin Market. I jumped as the phone interrupted my gloomy thoughts.

"Miss Baba," a curt voice said. "Miss McLennan would like to speak to you, please hold for a moment."

I froze. Butterflies stormed my stomach and a familiar tasting bitterness seeped upward to my throat.

"Miss Baba, you left so fast we could not tell you our decision," the hollow nasal-toned voice said. "We will admit you. You will be on probation and, if you pass the first semester, you will remain."

I covered the phone as I squelched a scream. "Miss McLennan, you won't be sorry," I told her. "I will do my best. I will be a success, you will see."

I hung up, stood and began to dance around the empty store, crying and laughing, saying, "thank you God!"

Thirty years later, in a hotel room, putting the finishing touches on my talk, I stopped in mid sentence. The California Board of Registered Nurses had asked me to speak at their state convention for nursing faculty and directors of nursing. The implications of what I was about to do began to take form.

I thought about my graduation on June 29, 1964 in Flint, Michigan. What would happen if I could take the faculty I was to speak to back with me to that auditorium? What if I could stand in front of myself and say, "Ruth Ann, do you know who I am and who's behind me?" What if I could go onto the stage and stand in front of Miss McLennan, and ask her the same question?

I smiled to myself because I'd come full circle—desire, flamed passion and focus. Is there any reason not to try when one knows they can?

Ruth Ann Obregon, RNC, MBA
Education Consultant, San Diego

"Be like a postage stamp.
Stick to something until you get there."
Josh Billings

Fifty Thousand and Counting

The crowd at the jam-packed ballpark was enthusiastically singing, "Take Me Out to the Ball Game." My husband and I, along with our two grandsons, were enjoying a balmy September evening watching the Los Angeles Angels of Anaheim. They had just scored and were now ahead by two runs. Five-year-old Ryan wanted to be lifted up so he could see over the standing crowd. I scooped him up, peanut shells falling from his shirt and pants. We sang in full voice and then laughed as we sat down at the end of the song.

"GUESS TONIGHT'S ATTENDANCE!" flashed on the scoreboard. The three choices were 45,617, 46,102 and 47,387.

"Wow! That's a lot of people," Sean, our 9-year-old grandson, exclaimed. Then it struck me like a thunderbolt! Just up the street, our Kaiser Permanente Anaheim midwives had delivered more babies than all the fans in this ballpark with a couple of thousand to spare.

Since L&D opened its doors at the Anaheim hospital on August 1, 1980, there has been a midwife present, 24/7, to provide care for women in labor and to deliver their babies. Our service has grown from three original midwives to the current 24, who also provide ongoing obstetrical and gynecological services for women of all ages in our offices.

Three days before the game, they called me in to cover L&D for Ilene, one of the original midwives hired when our service first opened. When I arrived, I found out that, after 27 years, our midwifery service was only three births away from delivering 50,000 babies. The unit was full of expectant mothers, so we knew the moment was close. Which baby would be our 50,000th? The atmosphere was ripe with excitement and anticipation.

Laura, the other midwife on duty, was attending a woman who was pushing with her first baby. We had already completed two deliveries. The 50,000 milestone was at hand. I was personally thrilled for Laura, because she had been one of my mentors in midwifery school, just as I was disappointed for Ilene who had been eagerly awaiting this moment.

Suddenly, L&D triage paged me. They had a woman who arrived in active labor and needed immediate evaluation. Minutes after settling mom and family into a birthing room, their second daughter, healthy and pink, announced her arrival with full voice. We were all exhilarated.

Then, one of the nurses said, "This is our 50,000th midwife delivery!" I could hardly believe it. Upon hearing the news, the family told us that they were long-time members and that many extended family members had been born at Kaiser Permanente. Hugs and tears mixed at this doubly miraculous moment.

After completing my paperwork, I pondered how I had ended up being part of such a momentous occasion. After all, I was the newest full-time member of the service, and only filling in for another midwife. But, this moment was not mine alone. This joyful milestone was the culmination of decades of dedication, service and commitment to our patients and their families. Our amazing group of midwives, teamed with wonderful physicians, nurses and techs, provides obstetrical care that far exceeds national standards.

At the stadium, Sean brought me back from my thoughts. "What do you think is the right answer, Grandma?" Looking around the colorful stadium filled with nearly 50,000 happy fans, my eyes welled up with tears. I could only say, "It sure is a lot of people!"

Cheryl Pearce, CNM, MSN
OB/GYN, Orange County

"We are miracles. Each of us is an absolute
astonishment. So whether you believe in
miracles or not, we still are.
We still partake of 'miracledom.' "
Ruby Doe

Groundhog Day

The 1993 movie "Groundhog Day" comes to mind each time I visit Euna. She answers the door wearing exactly the same clothing she wore on the last visit and she repeats the same stories over and over. I know I've heard each one dozens of times, but she tells them to me as if it's the first time.

Euna is a delightful, 91-year-old lady who lives alone in her condominium with her two cats. She has no living relatives and a neighbor serves as her primary caregiver. She came into the palliative care program a year ago because of her declining cardiac status. Her primary care physician thought that Euna would soon be appropriate for hospice care, but her condition hasn't changed much during the year.

During my visits I monitor her medications, fill her pillboxes and order refills for her, and instruct her on safety issues. I call her when there are extreme weather conditions to make sure she's warm or cool enough; and I called her when we recently had an earthquake because I knew she was home alone. Due to her forgetfulness, she needs frequent reminders in order to continue to live on her own.

Most importantly however, I listen to her stories. She loves telling me about how Johnnie Cat lost his tail when a car hit him, and about the truck driver that picked him up and dropped him off at the vet's office. She always gets teary when she remembers her other black and white cat, Bandit, who had to be put to sleep, but cheers right back up when she tells me how the vet gave her Johnnie as a replacement. "He was also black and white," she says.

Then she talks about how she found Sadie Cat cowering in the bushes during a rainstorm when Sadie was just a tiny kitten. "Sadie would probably have died that night if I hadn't found her," she tells me.

I love hearing Euna's stories and she enjoys recounting them. Sometimes I think senile dementia isn't such a bad thing, as long as there are patient people around to listen to the same tales again and again.

But then there are the days when Euna retells the story of her husband's sudden death at the breakfast table fifteen years earlier. "It was on July 5," she says each time. To Euna it is fresh in her mind and she is still grieving as though it happened yesterday. I feel pain in my heart for her as she cries over her loss. And then she talks about her daughter whose death was just five years ago.

Sue was her only child. She had married briefly and was childless. Sue had turned to alcohol to ease her life's pain and ultimately died of an alcohol-related illness. Her daughter's death hurt Euna even more than suffering the loss of her husband. "There's no way to settle losing your child before you," she always says. Being the last one left alive is almost a fate worse then death in her eyes.

So I continue my weekly visits which Euna looks forward to and remembers because she writes them on her calendar. I don't know how many times I will hear her stories. When they stop, I will surely miss them and Euna, too. But, I will know that Euna is finally at peace, and hopefully with her lost daughter and husband on the other side.

Kathy Pratt, RN, BSN, PHN
Hospice, Bellflower

"Since you cannot do good to all, you are to pay special attention to those who, by the accidents of time, or place, or circumstances, are brought into closer connection with you."

Augustine of Hippo

I Will Always Keep You
in My Prayers

Three years ago I cared for Steve, a 57-year-old male suffering from congestive heart failure and uncontrollable diabetes. He was on two liters of oxygen. As a man weighing 334 pounds, his swollen legs made it difficult getting out of bed and he needed assistance.

The outgoing shift told me that Steve refused to accept help from his family and I did not understand why. His family was willing to assist him until he recovered. The discharge planner even gave him a list of resources but he continued to decline help.

As I walked towards Steve's room, I thought of using the caring model. When I entered, the expression on his face told me that he was deeply troubled and had a lot on his mind. I introduced myself, sat beside him and began to converse with him hoping to get his mind off whatever was bothering him.

I found out that Steve had just retired after 34 years of federal service, six years in the U.S. Army Medical Department and 28 years in the Department of Veterans Affairs, Health Care Administration. As an unmarried man, he spent most of his life depending on no one but himself, doing everything on his own, and taking pride in his independence. He was not used to relying on others and so in his current situation, he refused the offered help from his family.

"I don't want to become a burden to them," he said.

"Steve, you must be blessed because you have a family who is willing to help you," I said to him. He then admitted that his struggle with pride hindered him from accepting his family's assistance.

"This is difficult for me to grasp," he said in a troubled voice. "But it is something that I have to figure out. I believe I have to pray to be humble."

As I gazed into his eyes, I asked him if I could say a prayer for him. Steve, with his eyes brimming with tears, nodded his head. I prayed that he would have the strength to put aside his pride and instead to be filled with humility as he faced his current situation.

Two months after Steve's discharge, I received a letter from him. It read:

> *Dear Melinda: I lost 40 pounds. I am slowly on my way to an ideal weight. My blood sugar is also now under control. Most of all, my family has been instrumental in my recovery. I will never forget your kindness, compassion and care at a difficult juncture in my life. Thank you again. God bless you!*
>
> *I will always keep you in my prayers. Steve*

There is a saying that goes, "A successful nurse can be measured not only in achievements, but in lessons learned, lives touched and moments shared along the way." Nursing is not always easy, but to have the opportunity to make a difference in someone's life is an unforgettable blessing that will last a lifetime.

Melinda Guran, RN, BSN
Medical-Surgical, Orange County

"Caring is the shining thread of gold that
holds together the tapestry of life."
Ida V. Moffett

For Eric

I spent my 25th birthday as an inpatient on what would later come to be called the Valley Medical Unit at Kaiser Permanente Fontana. I was five-months pregnant with my second child and admitted with complications. To be perfectly frank, I was feeling ashamed for complaining of pain. Jeanne, my dear sister-in-law and friend, was battling a cancer that would soon take her life. She suffered daily with pain and nausea, yet she never uttered a complaint.

What right did I have to gripe? I would recover from an illness that would be a memory in a few short days; Jeanne herself would be a memory in a short matter of time.

Missing my 22-month-old son drained me emotionally. Again, there was the element of shame. At least I could expect to see him grow into manhood. Jeanne would not know the joy of watching her daughter become a lovely woman.

Then along came my nurse Eric. The first time I met him, I was buried in my blankets, curled into a fetal position, crying. He simply announced he was there to help with whatever I needed. He pulled a chair up next to the bed.

"I'm here if you want to talk," he said and then just sat there.

I really wanted to get rid of him so I could continue my pity party, but he just wouldn't leave. After a time, I emerged from my self-made cocoon and confided that I was ashamed for feeling sorry for myself. He gently smiled, reached out, took my hand and said, "What makes you think that being sad, lonely and in pain is something shameful?"

He then encouraged me to talk about Jeanne, my son and my feelings. Eric's quiet support and non-judgmental attitude made it okay to expect relief from physical and emotional pain. Eric made sure I understood that nurses do not judge a patient's emotional state or compare them one to another.

"Each person experiences illness in their own unique way," he told me.

He routinely administered analgesia with a healthy helping of compassion and humor. He conspired with my husband and family to smuggle my son in the back door for a visit. After all, hospital visiting was strictly regulated. He then kept my little boy plied with Jell-O so the nursing supervisor wouldn't hear him and find out about the indiscretion.

Each time he entered or left my room, he reached out, sometimes a simple pat on the shoulder, other times a soft handshake but always with a sense of human-to-human caring. During those evening shifts, Eric became more than a nurse, he became a shining inspiration.

A few months later, after the birth of my second son, I returned to school. I felt passionately that when Eric held my hand, he handed me a relay torch. It was now my turn to carry it forward and enlighten others' lives.

I had hoped to someday tell him what a difference he made, not only in my life at a time when I needed acceptance and care, but in the life of each patient I have touched through 25 years of nursing. Sadly, I never met him again. I only hope he knows what a difference he made by sitting down, reaching out and holding my hand.

Joyce Piper, RN, BSN
Department Administrator, Hospital Nursing, 4 East, Fontana

*"The true meaning of life is to plant trees
under whose shade you do not expect to sit."*
Nelson Henderson

Feline Fiasco

Paul was an older man who lived alone in a second-floor apartment. Actually, Paul didn't live alone; he had two cats, ages 15 and 17, who had been devoted companions.

When Paul came into our hospice program, he was thin, weak and needed to be in a nursing home. But he refused to leave until I found a home for his cats. For two weeks, I ardently researched various options. The cats' ages definitely made it a challenging task.

Finally, the day came. Paul had to leave and his ill daughter would have to find a home for the cats. But on my last trip to see Paul, I forgot to bring the necessary forms. When I returned to the office to retrieve them, the phone rang. Hallelujah! A home was found for the felines!

Paul agreed to leave that day and said the neighbors in the adjacent upstairs apartment had a key that I could use the next morning to get the cats. Not so! When I arrived the next morning, I found one cat outside, the other inside and no key!

Instantly distressed and desperate to find a way into his apartment, I decided to call his hospice case manager for ideas. Luckily, she knew that Paul's front balcony door was always unlocked.

It was no easy feat coaxing two felines into travel carriers. The older stubborn one did a Houdini escape instantly. It was a half-hour before persuasion, sweet talk and some not so sweet talk, fast action and food got him back into the carrier.

All the way to the drop-off point, I spoke to the cats in their carriers in the back seat as if my words could provide logic and counsel for them in their noisy distress. I must have looked crazy. When we arrived, the real moment of emotion exploded. I cried with the cats, thinking about the changes and losses we all faced.

Paul was content in his new home. I continued to visit him. The couple who had his pets sent pictures for me to give to Paul. The cats looked well adjusted. It was a moment of peace and release for Paul who died two months later.

Paul is still in my heart and yes, so is the memory of his two old cats.

Vicki Smurlo, MSW
Wilshire Hospice, Los Angeles

"I love cats because I love my home and after awhile they become its visible soul."
Jean Cocteau

Over the Crowd Came a Voice

One incredible day a few years ago, my husband Mark and I were at the Bradley International Terminal at the Los Angeles International Airport. We were seeing our Japanese exchange student off on her return trip home. This was a momentous occasion and my camera was ready to capture every minute of her journey for pictures to send to her later.

Suddenly, I heard my name called from the upper level. Mark told me that I must be crazy and could not possibly have heard my name in the middle of a massively crowded airport terminal. But, there it was again, "Ilene!" I quickly scanned faces for one I would know. Lo and behold, there she was, Leah, one of my patients with her entire family waving at me. I realized in an instant that, lined up in order of age, were all five of the children that I had cared for in utero and those I had delivered. I immediately raised my camera and took that special photo which hangs in my office to this day.

A few minutes later, we were reunited, right in the middle of the hubbub that was going on around us. I think we were all equally astonished by the coincidence, a standout moment. There were hugs all around before we parted ways. I think I smiled all the way home!

There are parts of my job that I don't like and would gladly retire from in a heartbeat. I am, after all, part of the over-60 crowd and I often wonder if it is the right time. Then I think about all the families whose lives I have touched and who have touched mine in my 27 years at Kaiser Permanente. I would surely miss my patients. I am now delivering the daughters of those women I delivered. I would certainly miss the sights, sounds and smells of birth, each one just a little more wondrous.

I am at a crossroads; thinking about retirement is tricky for me. I am, after all, just 63 deliveries away from my 5,000th Kaiser Permanente Anaheim baby. Delivering my last baby will be heart wrenching. How will I watch that child grow? Many families keep in touch with pictures and updates, and that yearly Pap appointment is far more than just a physical exam, tests and charting.

For 42 years, I have been a practicing nurse, the last 30 years as a certified nurse-midwife. I am the senior midwife at Kaiser Permanente Anaheim. It is who I am and who I was always meant to be. I am linked by my experience, my connections and my journey. Retirement cannot take those things away, especially not stories like that day at the Bradley International Terminal.

Ilene Gelbaum, CNM
Senior Midwife, OB/GYN, Orange County

"A new baby is like the beginning of all things—
wonder, hope, a dream of possibilities."
Eda J. Le Shan

Cheat Sheets

I started my nursing career at Kaiser Permanente in March 1984. I was introduced to a new field of nursing practice, telephone nursing. At the time, no one recognized it as a specialty. As we took calls, we filled out forms with the caller's main issue. Being new, I tried to find articles and books that would help me in my work. I could find very little.

Eventually, I put together a "kardex" and called it my "cheat sheets." I would jot down appropriate questions to ask along with some red flags. For example, along with the usual questions, if the caller had abdominal pain, I wanted to be sure to ask a female of childbearing age about her last period and what contraceptive method she was using. When a caller had upper abdominal pain, I wanted to be sure that I considered cardiac-related questions. With one call after another, I found it easier to focus and be more thorough if I had something handheld that I could refer to quickly.

Over the years, these cheat sheets would grow. Often my peers would ask to use them and even contribute to them. I was delighted that they would share their expertise. They would also encourage me to write a book. Me? Write a book? In my dreams!

The years went by and my kardex got bigger. I read whatever I could about telephone nursing. There was not much. During my research, I would come across articles that would warn of the dangers of telephone triage and describe very poor outcomes with resultant litigation. My heart would ache. After reading the details, I would add additional information to my kardex notes to enhance the telephone interview process.

In 1992, I completed my master's thesis on "The Effects of a Nursing Process Oriented Form on Documentation of Nursing Interventions among Telephone Triage

Nurses." I discovered through my literature search that there was still not much written about telephone nursing. Then, it hit me like a ton of bricks! I had worked in the field longer than anyone who was publishing anything on the subject.

My kardex was a system that I had developed over the years. I felt comfortable using it and it had input from my peers, who were all experienced expert nurses in various areas. It also contained information from reviews of actual litigation. What a wealth of information! How helpful it would be to share it with other nurses also struggling to do their best.

I suddenly felt a strong calling to contribute to the knowledge base on telephone nursing practice and started to develop a continuing education course for nurses. I gave local seminars, sometimes with a friend of mine who was an attorney. There were always lots of questions about litigation.

I found nurses were very eager to learn whatever they could and very concerned that they might miss something in the conversation with the caller. Getting out and listening to other nurses gave me more energy and passion. I always learned so much from them! I also started work on a book for nurses. It would be like the kardex, a flip chart for quick reference with bullets for red flag items. It took two years to complete.

I sent query letters to about ten publishing companies and then I waited. The nursing editor from Mosby called. She wanted to talk to me about a book contract. I was on cloud nine! Now, I had deadlines to meet. I would wake up early on the days I devoted to writing and could not believe it was already dark by the time I glanced out of the window. I guess writers call this "flow." I had unbelievable energy and required little sleep. When the book was nearing completion, Kaiser Permanente physicians and nurses who were experts in their fields graciously volunteered as consultants to review it before publication.

"Telephone Health Assessment—Guidelines for Practice" came out in 1996. After publication, I went on book tours across the country. I did seminars and got to speak to thousands of nurses. I traveled from New York, Baltimore, and Boston to Atlanta, New Orleans, and up to St. Louis and Cleveland. It was the most exhilarating experience of my professional life! I learned that nurses are the same all over. We love to learn, we all want to do our best and we all care very much about our patients.

And, boy do we have stories!

It has been many years and telephone nursing has become a certificated specialty. Now there is a wealth of information and some very sophisticated and expensive computer programs available. The second edition of my book came out in 2001 but I still feel like a pioneer. I was so blessed by the people who offered their expertise, support and encouragement, and held me up through the rough times, and yes, there were those! Contributing to the body of knowledge and assisting other nurses in their journey to provide quality telephone health assessments has been an indescribably awesome experience. I feel so lucky that I have had the opportunity to pursue my passion and live the dream!

Sandi Anderson, NP, MSN
OB/GYN, Orange County

"I never lose an opportunity of urging a practical beginning, however small, for it is wonderful how often the mustard seed germinates and roots itself."
Florence Nightingale

In the Land of Cowboys

In the land of cowboys and large steak houses with neon lights lived a young man known as the "at least kid." He had an inspiring soul. Despite his age and despite the cards life dealt to him, he always saw the sunny side of things. For him all things could have been worse. He accepted his fate with dignity; his only request was that we would remember him as the "boy named Griffin" who was brave and who did everything to fight the "bad guys."

I was packing and preparing to visit Griffin who had moved to Texas. You see, I had the privilege of caring for Griffin at a local children's hospital. Most people would not think of it as a privilege to care for and grow very close to a 5-year-old boy fighting neuroblastoma; but if you knew him, you would absolutely understand. He touched many lives, making more of a difference than most people who live ten times the number of years he lived.

Two days before I was to arrive in Texas, Griffin's mother Monique had to have one of the most difficult conversations that a mother would ever have to have with her child. It was in January 2005 when she had to tell her son that they had lost their fight with the "bad guys."

"Mom, can't we go to a different hospital? Can't we see a different doctor?" he'd said. "Isn't there anything else? I don't want to die."

Monique's heart was broken. She had to tell him there was nothing left that any doctor could do. She told him how much she loved him and let him know that he had done everything he could do.

"At least I can go to heaven and not feel sick and I can see all my friends—Paige, Ryan and Courtney," Griffin answered. That was always Griffin's response to any bad news; "at least" followed by the brighter side of things.

Two hours after Griffin's conversation with his mother, I received a phone call. It was Griffin telling me that he would not be able to see me when I arrived in Texas, that he loved me, and that his trip to heaven was going to be the best trip ever.

Griffin stayed awake all night calling those he loved to say goodbye. When he died that early morning in January 2005, he was barely 6 years old. I awoke suddenly, knowing he had just passed. His mother said that everyone he called that night shared the same story—of waking up at the same time he had died.

Dear Griffin: Thank you for teaching me to love life, and to see things through rose-colored glasses. Most importantly, thank you for reminding me that a hundred years from now it will not matter what my bank account contained, what sort of house I lived in, or the kind of car I drove. But the world may be different because 'at least' I was important in the life of a child, especially yours.

Love always, Debbie

Debra Lynne Robb, RN, MSN
Education, Panorama City

"How wonderful it is that nobody need wait a single moment before starting to improve the world."

Anne Frank

GRID to AIDS,
One to Two

I remember the early days of the AIDS epidemic as if they were yesterday. Of course, no one called it AIDS then. First, it didn't have a name. Then we called it GRID, gay-related immunodeficiency, because every patient we saw was a gay male.

So many nurses were frightened. We didn't know what this mysterious disease was or how it spread. But we did know that these men were extremely sick. They were febrile and weak. Some had almost intractable diarrhea, which meant that they needed a great deal of nursing care for which one needed to totally gown, mask and glove.

The numbers and acuity of these patients started to take their toll on the nurses caring for them. Because we considered them "heavy patients," we assigned them from one nurse to the next nurse every day. I recognized that part of the difficulty of caring for these patients was the sense of helplessness and isolation that the nurses felt in the rooms. Our lack of understanding of what was going on and the great effort it took to engage the patients in conversation compounded the issues.

I proposed a pilot to "double-assign" these patients to two nurses each day. This meant that two nurses were well acquainted with the status and needs of the patient, and they could easily take turns answering the call light. When baths and linen changes needed doing, the nurses could go in together. Having two nurses in the room lifted everyone's mood. It was easier to engage the patient in conversation, to reflect on and address the patient's fears as well as introduce lighthearted banter when that was appropriate too.

This scenario is over 20 years old, yet I still remember the impact of this pilot. Our patients responded very well to having two nurses each day. Rather than make them feel like a burden, they felt special. But the effect on the nurses was noticeable as well. It was a great lesson on teamwork and on mitigating the most difficult of circumstances when nurses collaborate and support one another.

Felice Klein, RN, MN
Director, Physician Education, Pasadena

"To each age comes its own peculiar problems and challenges, but to it also comes the necessary vision and strength."
Ruth Weaver Hubbard

Two Big-Hearted Brothers

My husband, Bruce Dufelmeier, was the 2007 Nurse of the Year at Kaiser Permanente Los Angeles and has just celebrated his 25th year of service in October. He spent most of that time working in the ICU, but for the last seven years he's found it more fulfilling to work in home health because he sees the difference he makes in the lives of patients.

* * * * *

One Thanksgiving Day, Bruce said, "Let's celebrate in a different way." So, with the patient's permission, he brought our kids and me along with him to the patient's apartment.

When we got there, we found the man living amidst trash and dirty dishes with clothes strewn all over the place. His wife lived in a nursing home. Friends picked him up sometimes so he could visit her.

Armed with big trash bags, we started cleaning and picking up. When we began, we couldn't see the carpet and there was no place to sit. Our family spent half a day and collected 16 big bags of trash. Later, I went to pick up some food and we had lunch together. The man was in tears.

* * * * *

Tom is in his 80s and Miguel, his partner, is younger but much sicker with diabetes. He needed a leg amputation. They live up in the hills of Silverlake. Tom can't drive anymore.

Bruce coordinated Miguel's trip to the hospital. When he got well, Bruce picked him up and brought him back to his home. Tom and Miguel invite us to every birthday. They are very appreciative.

* * * * *

Gary has a rare condition called Stiff Person's disease. He gets extremely anxious if a different nurse comes to him. He wants everything the same and he will wait until Bruce can see him. So, Bruce always squeezes him into his busy schedule even on his day off or while on vacation.

* * * * *

Bruce's brother, Tim Dufelmeier, is an ER nurse and has been Nurse of the Year at Los Angeles County Hospital for two years.

In the mid-90s, a disgruntled patient shot an ER doctor. As the doctor slumped over the table, Tim grabbed a gurney, loaded him onto it and took him to the operating room. The shooter watched the whole thing, still holding the smoking gun.

Tim shook all over after realizing that at that time, the doctor had a 5-year-old daughter. She is now grown. She wrote a very touching letter to my brother-in-law. "If it were not for you," she wrote, "I would have grown up without a dad."

There are many more stories to tell about both brothers. I have often congratulated my mother-in-law for giving birth to two wonderful sons who have big hearts.

Irma V. Dufelmeier, RN, CCRN
Acute Dialysis, Los Angeles

"To do what nobody else will do,
in a way that nobody else can do, in spite of
all we go through; is to be a nurse."
Rawsi Williams

Who Can You Be?

To some you'll be hope
To others strength.
A voice in the silence
A light in the dark.
A hand to hold
Someone to comfort.

Just who can you be?

With some you'll share joy
With others grief.
An encouraging word
A listening ear.
A sad goodbye
A newborn's cry.

My, who can you be?

Some days you'll feel glad
And others drained.
A smile for the healed
A shoulder for tears.
A halo shines
An angel disguised.

You're a nurse you see.

Gail Lindsay, RN, MA
Managing Director, Clinical Program Development
SCPMG Clinical Operations, Pasadena

Lost and Found

Friday was the big day, the Christmas party at the Braille Institute. It was also the last day of my community service rotation through the Kaiser Permanente School of Anesthesia. I had prepared for the day earlier in the week and I knew how important the celebration was for everyone, students and staff alike.

In the morning, they assigned me to the jazz band. I had a great time. The band was completely blind and they blew my mind. They were better than any jazz band I had ever heard. I danced with the students. They swept me off my feet and wore me out. Afterwards, I served lunch.

Catching my breath, walking towards the cafeteria, I ran into an old friend. It took a minute and then I realized I had graduated from Loma Linda University Nursing School with her in 1999. I hugged her and reintroduced myself.

"Oh, yes I recognize your voice," she said. "How are you? Are you here studying for your NP?" I told her my goals of becoming a CRNA and my school status. I told her it was my last day volunteering and, assuming she was studying for a higher degree as well, asked how much longer she would be working at the Braille Institute.

Instead she said, "I am a student here. I started losing my sight shortly after we graduated from nursing school. I am learning how to do regular, daily activities of life. I am now almost completely blind."

I think in nursing, or maybe in any profession that deals with tragedy, we become a little numb, but her answer affected me more than anything I could recall. Tears filled my eyes. Then, she said, "I know, what a waste huh?"

I hugged her and stupidly, without thinking said, "Are you okay?"

She smiled and said "I have to be, right? But I love this place and they are like family now. They are working with me and I have made so many friends here."

She explained to me that she has the inherited disease of retinitis pigmentosa. The photoreceptor cells in her retinas were continuously degenerating, causing cell death of the rods and cones in her eyes.

One more time she smiled and said, "Life is still good. I have my family, my education, and I have this place." I wished her luck and took my place in the serving line, scooping up potatoes and passing out corn bread.

My friend sat with the other students, laughing and having a good time. She looked so much as if she belonged there. But watching her brought back memories of our nursing class eating lunch together on the grass at school. I have to admit it took great strength not to cry all over the potatoes.

I knew the Braille Institute would give me great insight into how others manage. When I ran into my friend, it was the holidays. My two kids had very long Christmas lists; my studies and lack of financial support consumed me. I found myself stressed out and hyper-focused; it was so easy to forget who I was and what I had.

Later I found out that they were working with my friend and trying to figure out different ways she could use her four-year nursing education despite her blindness. Sometimes I forget how to be happy. But my friend was happy and strong despite her disease. My week at the Braille Institute and my friend gave me perspective which I needed.

Shannon Pfrunder, SRNA

Kaiser Permanente School of Anesthesia, Pasadena

"We could never learn to be brave and patient
if there were only joy in the world."

Helen Keller

What Baby Jared Taught Me

I first met Jared and his mom when he was admitted for sedation to have an MRI. Jared was 3 months old. He had a large growth on one of his feet, which his doctors had diagnosed as a hemangioma, but it was getting larger so they needed to do more tests. He was sedated, the procedure was completed and he was discharged home.

A month later, they were back. Jared had been to several specialists and a biopsy showed the growth as cancer. His parents were in shock, yet they had faith beyond anything I had ever seen. They shared with me their trust that God would heal their baby if it was meant to be and they had a strong belief that God would be with them throughout this ordeal. Jared's prognosis was very poor and few infants with this type of cancer survive.

Jared underwent chemotherapy treatments. He did amazingly well, little vomiting, few side effects, and as long as his mom was with him, he was happy. Above all, the tumor was disappearing! We were all amazed at how well he responded. They had told us the chemotherapy might not even stop the cancer from growing and now it was almost gone.

Jared, his parents and siblings spent lots of time rejoicing in this miracle. They gave credit to God for all of it. My faith too had grown in witnessing their complete trust and Jared's healing.

Now though, because he had responded so well to chemotherapy, the idea of doing a bone marrow transplant was recommended to his parents. The procedure might be his only chance for true long-term survival, but was not without very severe risks, including death.

His parents struggled for weeks with this decision. Their baby looked so normal. He had no tumor and no apparent cancer anywhere. Would it last? The transplant needed to be done before any tumor returned. They wanted to give him every chance to grow up.

With much prayer, they decided to proceed. He underwent the pre-transplant work-up including labs, X-rays, CTs and MRIs to make sure no cancer was present. He was cleared and the date was set.

A few days before he was to go to City of Hope to begin the transplant process, Jared could not move his legs and he was in obvious pain. An MRI showed tumors all along his spinal column. It had been less than two weeks since his last MRI that showed nothing.

I grew very angry. Why give this family such hope? Why give them a glimmer of survival just to take it all away? I shared my feelings with his mom. She was the voice of reason.

She believed this twist was a blessing. It was God's way of sparing Jared from the difficult procedure. God had spared her too. Had Jared not survived the transplant she would have struggled with her decision for the rest of her life. The decision was out of their hands. God had decided for them and they had peace in that belief.

Jared died a week later, at home, in bed with his parents. I joined them soon after. We bathed him and prepared him for the mortuary. His family was at peace, very sad, but at peace.

Since then, Jared's mom and I have kept in touch. We've spent time together and she's thanked me and all the other nurses for all the care, support and encouragement we provided her baby and her family over the six months of treatment and since his death.

But actually, I was the one who truly benefited from knowing this family. Their unfaltering belief in God taught me so much about commitment, trust and God's love. Through them, my faith is stronger than ever.

Lisa Kanady, RN
Pediatric Oncology, Fontana

"Without faith, nothing is possible.
With it, nothing is impossible."
Mary Mcleod Bethune

Spirituality, Healing and Nursing

It was one of those weekend night shifts when I wished I wasn't scheduled to work 12 hours on a critical care unit. I wanted to be at home with my family rather than going to my job. But my commitment to my patients and an obligation to fulfill my responsibilities strongly prompted me to be at work.

I was given the report on Mrs. Thompson, my 64-year-old patient with a diagnosis of asthma exacerbation. She had been extubated early on during the day shift and had been very anxious and uncomfortable. Sedation was ordered but could only be given in minimal doses because of her unstable respiratory status. I was also told that she had not been sleeping since she was in the unit, and was easily awakened and disturbed by even a slight touch or noise.

I made rounds and I introduced myself to her. I informed her that I was her night nurse. She was quiet and seemed to be resting. The first part of the evening was uneventful until half past midnight, when Mrs. Thompson's cardiac monitor alarm went off. It displayed a rapid heart rate but the O_2 saturation showed within normal limits.

I immediately went to check on Mrs. Thompson and found her very restless with labored breathing. I checked her vital signs. Her cardiac monitor was showing a heart rate greater than 100 beats per minute but with a normal rhythm. Her oxygen was on and her pulse oximetry was reading at 94 percent.

I put my arm around her, held her hand and asked if she was scared. She nodded her head slightly and in between breaths, she said "yes." I instructed her to do pursed lip breathing which she did. I could sense her apprehension and fear. I told her that

I would stay with her. It was at that moment that I thought of trying something I had never done in the many years of my nursing career. I took a big step.

"Would you like me to pray with you?" I whispered into Mrs. Thompson's ear.

"I would like that," said Mrs. Thompson without a second of hesitation.

I grasped her hand tightly and invited her to join me as I offered prayers for her healing, comfort and reassurance. I uttered my simple words fervently and surrendered Mrs. Thompson's fears, concerns, worries and pain to God. I prayed for her to have the strength and the willpower to get better and to entrust herself to the will of the Almighty.

I must have prayed with Mrs. Thompson so intently that I did not even hear the sound of the cardiac monitor. The stillness of the moment and the quiet surrounding us, in spite of the normally noisy ICU environment, was unusual. It was as if the world had stopped turning for a moment. All I heard was the sound of Mrs. Thompson's breathing.

I looked up at the monitor and noted that her heart rate had come down and displayed a normal sinus rhythm. Her O_2 saturation continued to display normal values and her breathing slowed down. Her facial expression looked relaxed and calm and her eyes appeared weary and sleepy.

Mrs. Thompson gratefully smiled at me and thanked me for taking the time to be with her and pray with her. She told me she felt much better. I gave her a dose of her ordered sedation, repositioned her in bed, gave her a back rub and made her comfortable.

I left her room at 1 a.m. trying not to disturb her so she could get that much-needed sleep. She must have slept soundly because even the pumping of the automatic blood pressure monitor on her arm did not bother her at all. It was 5 a.m. when Mrs. Thompson turned on her call light. I went to her room to find out what she needed.

"That was the best sleep I've had in four days," was the first thing she said. "Thank you so much for what you have done to help me and for being my nurse."

Her words created a remarkable moment in my professional life. I had never in my over 30 years of nursing used spiritual intervention in caring for my patients. Belief and trust in God as the most powerful healer was always a part of my personal life but I did not want it to interfere with my patients' own spiritual beliefs. But that night, I felt the need to do more for Mrs. Thompson. I sought intervention beyond my clinical ability, something that I knew only God could do, heal her body, mind and spirit.

I used to focus only on the physical aspect of the care I provided to my patients. But my experience with Mrs. Thompson brought me to a new high point and gave me a broader perspective on how I deliver my nursing care.

To make a person whole again, it takes healing both the body and the spirit. Since Mrs. Thompson, prayer has come to be a valuable element in the way I plan and provide care for my patients. Truly, my faith is one of my precious blessings.

Cecile P. Jalandoni, RN, MN, CCRN, CNS

Project Manager III, Ambulatory Clinical Practice, Orange County

"More things are wrought by prayer than this world dreams of."

Alfred, Lord Tennyson

Ceremony

In memory of Marie Cowan

Ceremony wasn't important to me at the age of 21.

In 1967, the University of California, Los Angeles (UCLA) held its commencement only once a year, in June. The departments and schools graduated together in one large, impersonal, very-hot-day-on-the-bleachers ceremony outside on the lawn where Drake Stadium stands today.

The Nursing Class of 1967 still had one awful summer quarter to go. Why go through the pomp and circumstance when graduation wasn't even official for us? So we didn't march in the ceremony—all 25 of us. There were no caps and gowns for the Class of 1967.

Ceremony wasn't important to me at the age of 26.

In 1972, UCLA still held graduation only once a year, in June. But, this time it wasn't an issue of impersonal, all of the schools together in one big track stadium. Now it was an issue of one big physical dilemma—my due date!

I was pregnant with my second child, hoping to get through the written portion of my comps, the oral portion of my comps, and not deliver before I had done both. They would never fail an $8\frac{1}{2}$-month-pregnant graduate student, would they?

So again, there was no cap and gown for this member of the Class of 1972 UCLA Graduate Nursing Program. Instead a bundle of joy named Lauren was born a week before commencement.

Ceremony gained importance to me at the age of 53.

One day, I found myself sharing with Marie Cowan, the Dean of the UCLA

School of Nursing, that despite my degrees from the school over which she now presided, and despite my associate faculty position for over 10 years—I had never donned the blue and gold hood (Bruin colors, of course) lined with apricot velvet (the conferring color for nursing) and marched in a processional university graduation. With that knowledge, Marie orchestrated a very special experience.

As is customary, only the Dean of a school can confer its degrees on its graduates. But Marie remembered her own daughter's graduation at the University of Washington some years before—where she was the faculty and her daughter was the graduate.

So an exception was made. Marie officially arranged the same special moment for me. On June 10, 1998, along with the Dean, I handed my daughter, Lauren, her Master's Degree in Nursing—cap, gown, tears and all!

Terry Bream, RN, MN
Administrator, Ambulatory Clinical Services, SCPMG, Pasadena

"While we try to teach our children all about life,
our children teach us what life is all about."
Unknown

Hector

I have always loved to help those people who may be sick or needy. I will always be glad to make a difference in the lives of my patients even if I have to go out of my way to help them. One true incident took place a few months back when I realized that even if we say a few words of inspiration and support to a sick person, it works and amazingly well.

Hector was a nurse at the University of California Irvine Medical Center with whom I had worked for a few years. He was a very handsome, well-built, soft-spoken and polite man. I knew his wife very well. I had seen him last when he became the father of a sweet little girl.

One day as I was getting off the elevator to report at work, I heard a familiar voice calling me. To my surprise, it was Hector's wife. She told me that Hector was a patient in the ICU. I immediately went with her to visit him. What I saw was tragic and shocking.

There lay Hector, unconscious, not knowing where in the world he was. While going to a fast-food place during his lunch break, a car hit him. The impact flung him 15 feet. He hit a wall, leaving him almost totally paralyzed. My emotions knew no bounds and I really wanted to cry.

Hector had not responded for days. I held his hand tight and said, "Hector! I am your friend Raj! You need to be strong and get out of your bed!" He tried to move his eyelids and I knew Hector would walk and run again.

His wife didn't want to remain in the room with him because it was hard for her to see him in this terrible state.

"Be strong," I told her. "Talk to him all the time. Tell Hector you love him and everything will be fine." Something changed after that day. His wife began to stay by his side. His family did the same.

I started visiting him every day. I would talk to him and help him in every way that I could. I knew he needed tender, loving care.

After a few days, Hector regained consciousness. He started getting better. I watched him improve each day. Finally, one day he was ready to go to a rehabilitation center. I always inquired about him. I was so pleased when I learned that Hector finally returned home.

I had an urge to see him personally. I met a mutual friend and learned that Hector was back to work. My joy knew no bounds. I thanked God for his speedy recovery. God works miracles and Hector was one of them.

Two days later, as I was discharging a patient, I thought I saw a familiar person sitting on a bench. To my great joy, it was Hector. I think God knew I wanted to see him. The same handsome guy who seemed almost dead was right there. I hugged him with tears in my eyes. At that point, I knew that I did the best I could for Hector.

I played a small role in his recovery that had its place along with the care he received in the hospital and the love and support of his family. Together we gave him the opportunity to live again!

Raj Chauhan, CNA
Definitive Observation Unit, Orange County

"Kindness in words creates confidence.
Kindness in thinking creates profoundness.
Kindness in giving creates love."
Lao Tzu

Monster

Dedicated to Martha Pascale, RN, the best,
a pioneering and idealistic spirit

My cat's name is Monster, so named by his former and now deceased owner, Carlton P. Edwards, who died of tongue cancer which rapidly spread to the throat and esophagus. Mr. Edwards was a long-time smoker and as he described himself, an "old drunk." I acquired Monster in May 1988.

I arrived at work early that day and was walking across our parking lot when I noticed an old large car packed to the hilt with sundry items. What a mess! It looked as if someone lived in it. I noticed an open ice chest full of water and scattered cat food.

Then I saw him, a cat living in that grubby car. His fur was pitch black and his body so thin. He was in the back seat that was crammed almost to the ceiling with stuff. I couldn't believe it. I said what I thought to be a few comforting words and left to tell the security guard.

"We know," he said. "He's been there for three days."

"But it has been hot," I said. "The window is open only a crack!"

The guard said, "You want a cat?"

I told him I already had two cats and three dogs. I asked him about the owner and found out he was on the fourth floor.

"That's my floor!" I said.

The elevator couldn't take me up fast enough. I had to do something about that cat! Questions flew through my head. Would my supervisor understand if I requested time off on such short notice? What would my husband say?

I quickly found out that the patient had tongue cancer and that it had spread to his throat. He was going to surgery at 9:30 a.m. to get a permanent tracheotomy and a feeding tube. I went to his room and saw a very thin man, looking much older than his 59 years.

As I entered, he looked at me. I went to his bedside and held his hand. I told him I was so very sorry and I asked about his cat. He said he didn't know what he was going to do with him since he would be in the hospital for some time.

"His name is Monster," he said. "I've had him since he was a kitten. He would run and bang into anything and everything."

"I'll take him if that's alright," I said.

"Okay, you can have him," he said.

Tears passed between us. Monster and Mr. Edwards had only each other. They had lived in his '63 Buick for over a year.

I went about my work that morning. My supervisor came in at 8:30 a.m. I explained everything, especially that Monster the cat needed to get out of that car before the inside temperature became too hot. She didn't know if anyone else would be available to work. My coworkers didn't seem to understand the urgency either.

At 10 a.m., I went out to the car and got in to check on Monster. There was only enough room for me to sit behind the steering wheel. The cat jumped into the back seat. He would not let me touch him. There was water and food for him.

When I went back to work after five minutes, some fleas accompanied me, easily seen on my white uniform. I continued to "bug" my supervisor until she agreed to find a replacement for me.

The discharge planner heard I was taking the cat and asked me if I was going to pay for the cat's expenses. I said yes. The social worker was very pleased, because the fate of Monster had bothered Mr. Edwards a great deal. They had scheduled the humane society to pick up his cat later that day. I felt like I was in a race against time.

At 2:30 p.m., the supervisor had all but given up on finding someone to come in to work early. I made a suggestion.

"I know Veronica would come in," I said. "She just got a cat. She'll understand the situation."

She did understand and came in right away. My workday ends at 4 p.m. Thanks to Veronica and my supervisor, I was able to leave at 2:45 p.m. I called my vet for an appointment. Then I contemplated how to get Monster out of the car he had lived in for over a year.

I parked my vehicle next to the '63 Buick, got in and talked to him. With my arm extended, I touched his nose. He was so happy that he somersaulted on his back and allowed me to caress him.

"Go for it now," I thought and grabbed him. I held tight and made it to my vehicle with only two scratches and several more fleas. During the nine-mile drive to the vet, he lay curled up in my lap. The next day I brought Monster home. It took a few weeks, but he finally adjusted.

I visited Mr. Edwards twice weekly in the nursing home and gave him a framed picture of his beloved pet. He was too weak to come and see Monster. When Mr. Edwards died two months later, he was so happy about his cat. He told a friend of his, "I found a good home for Monster."

I had Monster for nearly nine years until he disappeared in March 1997. He was about 10 years old. That cat loved me. I was the only one in my family he liked. Not a day goes by that I don't think of him. I miss that Monster.

Heidi Lehmann, RN
Family Medicine, South Bay

*"No amount of time can erase the memory of a
good cat, and no amount of masking tape can
ever totally remove his fur from your couch."*
Leo Dworken

A Dot of Blessing

I met a little person named Dot one day. Well, actually I met his mom and dad. Dot wasn't his real name, just the nickname that they gave him after their very first ultrasound showed a "dot" with a heartbeat, a heartbeat already in sync with theirs.

Dot was growing so well, just being 22 weeks into his development. He weighed a little over a pound and showed all the signs of a healthy and normal neonate. Unfortunately, his home environment sprung a leak and he was now in great jeopardy.

There was no way he could stay where he was because current conditions would not allow him to grow and develop safely. He would only have a 1 percent chance to live and his mother would probably get very sick too. The other choice was to allow the doctors to evict him; losing the 1 percent he and his family were clinging to.

When his mom and dad heard the news, they sobbed at the possibility that Dot's home might never be restored. Their tears resonated throughout the unit. Regardless of the controversy of when a fetus is a life, that night it was obvious a life was threatened, and everyone on the unit felt it.

For four days, we watched and cared for Dot and the family, doing everything medically to promote health. Mom was kept in bed with her legs slightly elevated to promote more fluid accumulating around Dot. Increased measures were taken to guard against infection since that was one of the greatest risks for both mom and baby.

Through several ultrasounds, we were able to see more fluid each day around little Dot. We could see Dot sucking a thumb or a toe and showing every sign of life. Our doctors fought to do all they could at the patient's request; however, her insurance provider denied further hospitalization.

She left in tears, touched by the care that she received. I hugged her goodbye with hopes that sometime in the future, I would look up and see her walking into our unit with Dot cradled in her arms.

Not all stories have a happy ending and yet all of them have a lesson to be learned. It took a little over four months before the ending of this story was told.

One busy night I was summoned to the phone. I apologized to my current patient and proceeded to answer the call.

"Hi, this is Karen, how can I help you?" I said.

The voice on the other end replied, "This is Tracy Adams. Do you remember me?"

"You are Dot's mom!" I quickly said, interrupting her mid sentence.

She sweetly acknowledged that she was and thanked me for remembering her. She told me that she lost Dot just one day after she left.

"Dot was a little girl," she said.

Before I could clear the tears of sorrow, she reassured me and explained she felt very blessed by this baby and blessed by the angels God had sent along the way because of her.

Dot had been cremated she told me. "I wear some of her ashes in a glass heart around my neck," she said. My tears flowed freely.

She had picked that very busy night four months later to call because it was her due date and rather than be sorrowful, she was calling to express gratitude and joy for all who cared for her and her baby. She said that God used all of us to bless her.

"Yes," I told her, "but God had also used you and Dot to bless all of us!"

Karen Perkins, RN
Labor and Delivery, Panorama City

"How far that little candle throws his beams!
So shines a good deed in a weary world."
William Shakespeare

Rewriting the Story of a Writer

At one time Kaiser Permanente operated their own SNFs. During this period, I was fortunate to teach at the SNF that served the South Bay, West Los Angeles and Los Angeles Medical Centers.

I had the daunting challenge of working with one of our patients who was a prolific writer with the Los Angeles Times. This patient had broken his neck and was now wheelchair bound. Our SNF had provided his rehabilitation.

He was nearly ready for discharge but still needed to learn how to do his own intermittent bladder catheterizations. Teaching his wife was not an option. Without this skill, the future looked dim for returning to his residence versus going to a permanent nursing home.

Fortunately, we had a great rehabilitation team at our SNF. With the help of the occupational therapist, a pair of prism glasses (special glasses that allowed him to look down without bending his neck) and the use of a floor-length mirror, we were able to train the patient to do his own catheterizations.

Initially, it was frustrating for the patient to learn how to orient his left from right images in the mirror, as well as relearning exercises to fine-tune his ability to grasp and hold himself steady to accomplish the procedure. It took two weeks and lots of patience and persistence. But we did it!

Happily, the patient was able to return to his own home and maintain his independence. This is one story out of many successes that reflected the outstanding care we provided to the patients who made their way to our SNF.

Barbara Hickman, CNS-Gerontology
Education and Training, Los Angeles

*"Anyone can look for fashion in a boutique or
history in a museum. The creative explorer
looks for history in a hardware store
and fashion in an airport."*
Robert Wieder

Room 3125

When I first started working in the ICU at Kaiser Permanente San Diego, I quickly realized how tragic life can be for some of our patients. Being a spiritual person, and struggling with the realities of critical care, I asked if anyone had ever witnessed what they would call a miracle. Most said no. We discussed how amazing it would be to personally experience such a thing.

Shortly thereafter, we had a 22-year-old male patient transfer to us from an outside facility. His story was one of those that make you wonder about life. He was young, strong, had a girlfriend, a loving family and a promising college degree in the works. His only medical issue was a surgically-corrected perspiration disorder.

He was hospitalized because he was up late playing basketball, became overheated and had a seizure that lasted for approximately 30 minutes. The paramedics intubated him in the field and transferred him to the closest hospital. Neurologists evaluated him, and diagnosed him with an anoxic encephalopathy, which is irreversible damage from lack of oxygen to the brain. His life was never going to be the same.

When he arrived on our unit, he needed to have a tracheostomy performed because of his prolonged dependence on a breathing machine. When I assumed care of him, discussions were in progress about long-term nursing homes. He would have to go to a facility that took care of ventilator-dependent patients. I was filled with sadness for the loss and uncertainty he and his family were experiencing.

I was his nurse for about three days. During that time, he was a one-to-one patient. He was extremely agitated and needed restraints. It was impossible to leave his bedside for fear that he would jump out of bed, injure himself or remove his tracheostomy. His family sat with him daily, able to do little but watch as he suffered through this awful experience.

At the same time, my wife, who was 32-weeks pregnant, began to have difficulties. She was admitted to the hospital and gave birth to my son Joshua three days later. Two days after his early delivery, I walked down to my unit to share the news with my coworkers. Out of the corner of my eye, I saw someone standing in the doorway of Room 3125. He was just starting to move and I had to adjust my eyes to confirm what I saw. There was my 22-year-old patient walking straight toward me, on his own, with his dad in tow.

In utter disbelief, I said his name. He stopped, looked up at me and stared into my face. His dad said, "This is John. He's one of the nurses who helped care for you."

This patient, who by all accounts had irreversible brain damage, opened his arms, stepped forward and gave me a hug. Through his speech valve he said, "Thank you for taking such good care of me." As I looked at the patient and his dad standing together, I thought of my newborn son and the gift of life, and was overcome with emotion.

I consider it a privilege to be a nurse. I have gained tremendous perspective through my ICU experience about the value of every single day of living. I will never forget my time in Room 3125, that hug, or that moment when I looked up and saw my patient standing with his dad. I had just experienced my very first medical miracle.

John Hoffman, RN
ICU, San Diego

*"I think miracles exist in part as gifts and in part as clues
that there is something beyond the flat world we see."*
Peggy Noonan

Welcome Sophia

It began when we were doing an epidural together in Birthing Room A. There were four Jennifers in the room: the nurse anesthetist, her CRNA student, the patient and myself! We all had a good laugh and tried not to get too confused!

Months later came the news that the nurse anesthetist, Jennifer, was, at long last, pregnant. She hoped that I could be there for the birth and I felt honored that she asked. You see, she is a very particular person, very detail oriented, with a terrific reputation among the nurses for a job well done when she places an epidural. Whatever she sets her mind to do, she does well.

Jennifer's due date came and went. Jennifer finally came in for induced labor. I took care of her on day two and at last got to meet her wonderful husband. He was so very attentive and easy to be around. On day three, the cervix was finally ready and we knew that this would be the long-awaited date! We were able to move to a birthing room and it was there that the mood was set. Jennifer had soothing instrumental music playing and the lights were low. It felt like a spa.

After the epidural, we turned Jennifer from side to side so the baby's head could labor down. Even when the pressure got extremely intense, her strength and resolve showed. True to her nature, she had thoroughly researched everything to help ease labor and had her husband find the human map of acupressure points that she had brought. With the acupressure, the breathing, the turning and the music, she was soon ready to push.

Tears of joy and love welled up in her husband's eyes as the pushing began. We fell into a rhythm of pushing and relaxing. The doctor stayed over to do the delivery and was pleased with her progress. At the end of my shift, I found that I could not leave this amazing couple.

With more controlled, forceful and steady pushing Sophia emerged, a brown-haired miracle! A beautiful girl with long eyelashes and the good fortune to be born loved and wanted into a very happy family.

I have been an L&D nurse for 23 years, but this delivery in particular made me remember why I chose my specialty and why the work we do is so important.

A family was born!

Jennifer F. Cordova, RN
Labor and Delivery, Fontana

"A child is a gift whose worth cannot be measured except by the heart."
Theresa Ann Hunt

Easter Sunday

I always thought that I could handle death and dying until I met Australia. He was 75 years old and critically ill.

It was Easter Sunday. Our minds are usually occupied with finding eggs and going to church. But, for me, those things were not in my thoughts, not on that day. The realization that Australia was going to die soon deeply affected me.

His daughter never left his side. I thanked her for being there with him. "Many people would rather not," I said.

"He is my dad and I want him to get better," she replied.

During my 12-hour shift, the daughter and I worked together along with the doctor to figure out what was next in his plan of care. Eventually, Australia stopped breathing and a Code Blue was called. We tried for a long time to bring him back. Those minutes felt like hours of desperation. His daughter never left the bedside.

I tried to be strong for her but the human in me was at a loss for words. I held her hand and she gave me a hug. We thanked each other for being there and finally the doctors pronounced him dead.

Sometimes words are not necessary to connect with others. The mere presence of compassion and love for another human being speaks louder than anything that could have been said. As we prepared him for the rest of the family, his eyes were closed and he finally looked relieved to be out of his agony and misery.

Whenever Easter Sunday comes along, I remember that day and think about what that holiday really signifies. Is it a day of Easter bunnies, egg hunts and candy? Maybe it is for some people. But for me, it is a day to be with family; a day to be with the ones you love through happiness and health or illness and death.

Teresa Cobian Alcala, RN
Relief Charge Nurse, 2300 Unit, South Bay

*"The best and most beautiful things in life
cannot be seen, not touched, but are
felt in the heart."*
Helen Keller

The Interview

Do you remember a pivotal job interview? Mine was in 1989, interviewing for an NP position at Kaiser Permanente San Diego. I felt unsettled when I returned home from the interview. I could not figure out what went wrong. I had prepared for the usual questions, I wore a conservative suit and sensible shoes. After all, I was interviewing with the orthopedic foot surgeon who would be my boss.

"I am sure he didn't like me," I said to my husband that evening. "All we did was argue. He kept harping on the differences between NPs and PAs. I doubt we'd make a good fit."

I chose to put the whole experience behind me. I am a firm believer that expertise is only half of a successful job. The other half of the job depends on good relationships with your colleagues. To my surprise, I got the job!

Fifteen years later, while I was out to dinner with that same orthopedic surgeon, I brought up that first interview, sharing my initial reaction and dismay with the encounter.

"I did it on purpose," he said. "I created the controversy to assess your reaction. I knew you would have to face disgruntled patients and physicians in the NP position. I needed to be sure you could stand your ground and articulate your position."

Over the years this physician had not only been my boss, he had become a mentor and a friend. He inspired and challenged me to do my best. I had the utmost respect for him and never wanted to let him down. Consequently, I always strived to improve my orthopedic skills and prepare for the orthopedic challenges I faced. As a mentor, he taught me the value of basing patient care decisions on scientific evidence.

"Verify the facts," he said challenging me to find the proof to support decisions for the required care of external fixator pins. I did. I embraced the concept of evidence-based practice.

Between 2004 and 2006, I along with three other orthopedic NPs from across the country, assisted in developing the first National Orthopedic Nurse Practitioner Certification Examination. Each one of the test questions and answers needed to be substantiated and then validated with documented evidence. I was thoroughly prepared for this task because at Kaiser Permanente San Diego we biannually update our orthopedic department protocols based on the review of the scientific and medical literature.

My mentor and first Chief of Orthopedics believed in me before I believed in myself, always finding the time to take advantage of a teachable moment. Many of those experiences started with the words, "Did I ever tell you about the time…?"

He invested his enthusiasm and energy in me along with numerous other employees and students who crossed his path. It was through his vision and risk taking that new graduate NPs were hired into the department that now includes three NPs and 14 PAs.

It was not uncommon for a group of us to go out for lunch always at his insistence and on his dime. Those informal gatherings generated collegiality, trust and warmth, and strengthened the department. We grew in our relationships with each other on a personal and professional level. He patiently sat through conversations about our child-rearing experiences as well as patient encounters. We lived through his joys as a grandparent, the sorrows of struggling with his wife's chronic illness and his struggle with ALS.

It has been a little over a year since Dr. Robert Colgrove's death. He touched us all by his love and passion for medicine, learning and his fellow man. I would not be the person I am had he not taken a chance and hired the first NP in orthopedics at Kaiser Permanente San Diego, and nurtured that role over the years with encouragement as well as challenges. As I contemplate his caring ways, I am inspired to continue the tradition to invest in relationships, personal as well as professional, that make up the fabric of my memories.

In preparation for this story, I spoke to Dr. Colgrove's daughter, Alexis Curtis, RN, PhD, who also happens to be an NP. "One of my dad's favorite aphorisms was 'Nobody cares how much you know, until they know how much you care,'" she said.

> *My dad firmly believed in the primacy of caring, supported by knowledge, competency, commitment and the ability to make and defend a decision. That is why he was an ardent believer in the contribution of NPs to the organization and that may help explain his somewhat unorthodox interview technique. Alexis :)*

Debra Palmer, NP
Orthopedics, San Diego

"Few things in the world are more powerful than a positive push. A smile. A word of optimism and hope. A 'you can do it' when things are tough."
Richard M. De Vos

Learning Cases

Ireceived the page in the early evening, just as the sun had gone down. At the time I was finishing the last days of my second ER rotation as an intern before transitioning back to the inpatient floors. I was thinking about how I had enjoyed ER work so much during my first rotation that I had chosen to do it again as an elective.

I liked the atmosphere; the ebb and flow of patient care and the diversity and number of cases. There were lots of learning opportunities for a young doctor eager to master the intricacies of formulating a diagnosis and treatment plan. It was exciting to carry out the procedures we rarely had a chance to perform as medical students—endotracheal intubations, chest tube insertions, central venous catheterizations, arterial line placements and cutdowns.

I enjoyed balancing the care of an adult going through a hypertensive crisis on one hand and a child experiencing an asthma attack on the other, MIs, acute abdomens, traumatic injuries and the quiet times in between suturing up small lacerations in the back room.

I answered the page in the ICU where it was relatively quiet. The lights were turned down. The patients were sleeping. Here and there, I could hear the soft whooshing of a ventilator. My sister-in-law answered the phone.

"They brought your dad to the hospital," she said.

While part of me was somehow able to continue conversing with my sister-in-law, another part of me was thinking about my father, 2,000 miles away, brought to the local hospital's emergency room by paramedics after suddenly collapsing in the bathroom.

I could picture him surrounded by doctors and nurses administering CPR. I imagined him intubated with various catheters and lines being placed into and onto his body while my mother, brother and sister watched helplessly nearby. The irony that the doctor in the family who was just finishing a second ER rotation, and who was just as helpless, was not lost on me. I prayed that he was not just a learning case for anyone.

My father passed away that night and patients ceased to be just learning cases for me.

Edwin L. Corpuz, MD
Psychiatrist, Behavioral Health, Panorama City

"This is my simple religion. There is no need for temples; no need for complicated philosophy. Our own brain, our own heart is our temple; the philosophy is kindness."
Dalai Lama

Only Nurses

Only nurses will return
Night after night
To sterile halls
Smelling of antimicrobials
The grief
The incremental healing
Where others may vomit
Or bleed
And make a general mess
On you
And yet still we return
Bringing hope in the door

Marilyn Mitchell, RN, BSN

Education Consultant, Education and Consulting Services, San Diego

General Wade

In the summer of my junior year of nursing school, I had a great opportunity to work at Georgetown University Hospital in the ER. I was looking for the chance, prior to my senior year of studies, to answer the question, "Is nursing the career for me?"

I worked 12-hour shifts both days and nights. I performed every possible task—assessments, chest compressions, catheterizations, IV starts, postmortem care and recording core temperatures. I saw small babies and the elderly, the very rich and the very poor, and the healthy to the deathly ill.

As I was ending one of my long 12-hour shifts, an ambulance arrived. Off rolled an elderly woman on a c-spine board and restrained for safety. The patient had fallen. No family accompanied her.

As soon as she hit the ER doors, everyone heard her. She was one feisty woman repeatedly shouting, "Get me out of this! I'm uncomfortable!" Her loud complaints required the best of the best in the ER to calm her down. Her needs demanded a swarm of professionals around her gurney.

Observing the situation, I chuckled. To me it was humorous to see one person cause such a ruckus. When her admission papers came, I was asked to band her and have her sign them.

I went to her cubicle. I looked at her name tag and asked, "Are you Helen Wade?"

"Yes," she responded with some huffiness. "I am the wife of the late General Wade."

I placed the armband on her. She pulled me close, looked straight into my eyes and asked, "Do you know who General Wade was?"

"No, sorry, I don't," I answered honestly knowing that American history was not one of my strong points. At the same time though, I was disappointed that I could not share this knowledge with her.

She looked at me very firmly, almost as if to scold me and said, "You should know."

Her way, her tone and her decisive nature was penetrating. My time with her was short, perhaps 30 seconds at most, but I felt bothered, almost burdened that I knew nothing about General Wade.

"Who is General Wade?" I asked another seasoned ER nurse before I checked out that evening.

"I have no idea," she said. "You shouldn't worry about it. People come through these doors who think they are famous and think you should know all about them." This was before the days of Google searches.

That night, after dinner, as my dad was rushing out the door to a business meeting, the burning question arose in my mind.

"Dad, who was General Wade?" I asked.

He froze in his steps; his face dropped. He turned and looked at me in total bewilderment. He began to stammer in his words.

"General Wade was your great uncle," he said. "He married your grandfather's sister Helen. She is the last living relative on the Morans' side."

General Wade was a great aviator and in 1924 he was part of a team that made the very first flight around the world. His airplane, that I would later see, is in the Smithsonian Air and Space Museum.

My dad was amazed and humbled at the unexpected encounter with my great aunt. The next day at work, I visited her in her hospital room. Throughout that summer, I made several visits to her home before she died.

This chance, 30-second encounter, this crazy twist of fate allowed me a friendship with the last living relative of my grandfather's family. It also taught me a few lessons.

My role as a student had put me in a place of discovery; as a result, I had an open mind. The seasoned, well-qualified ER nurse had passed this person's comments off as nonsense. To me, this old woman was my patient for 30 seconds, but she was also my teacher. Instinctively, I knew that to learn from this patient and understand her needs, I had to find out about General Wade.

This seemingly cranky individual passed onto me a piece of information that identified not only who she was but also who I am.

Professionally, I knew, in that revealing moment, that nursing was the best career for me. I learned, in that instant, that nursing is the art of treating every patient and every situation with dignity and respect.

On a personal level, I sometimes think about what would have happened if I had disregarded that 30-second encounter. If I had categorized it as nonsense I would have never known about General Wade, my great aunt Helen and about my family heritage. Listening and caring about her past unexpectedly revealed a part of my family history.

Marthie Baker, RN, BSN, MA
Westminster Pediatrics, Colorado

"Chance is always powerful. Let your hook
be always cast; in the pool where you least
expect it, there will be a fish."
Ovid

Worth the Effort

I walked into the exam room and on the table sat a slim, middle-aged woman. She was looking down at her hands. As I started to introduce myself, she began to cry. I don't usually have this effect on my patients so naturally I knew she was concerned with something very important. I placed my hand on hers and gently asked, "Wanda, what is it that you are so worried about?"

"I don't want to die,' she said through her tears. "They told me I needed to start insulin and that means I am going to die."

"Whoa," I said. "You are not going to die from starting insulin. Let's back up a bit and talk about a few things before we do anything, okay?"

"Okay" she sniffed.

"First of all, tell me about yourself," I said.

For the next 20 minutes, we went over her history with diabetes. We talked about what she liked to eat, when she was eating and what medications she was taking. We discussed how diabetes works in the body and the meaning of her lab results.

She was already on the maximum doses of her oral medications and had an A1C (which shows one's average blood sugar for a three-month period) of 14. In a person without diabetes, it runs from 4.5 to 6.5. I explained that this meant that her average blood sugar, day in and day out, was running about 450.

I moved closer and looked directly into her eyes as I started the dreaded conversation about insulin.

"Insulin is not your enemy," I said. "In fact most people with diabetes do not start insulin early enough to prevent the problems caused by high blood sugar. May I show you how it is given; how easy it is to do? Then we'll see if you can try it just once a day, okay?"

She looked very anxious but she agreed. I walked out and came back in with a vial of saline and a syringe. I took her through the process of drawing up the "insulin" and reading the dose. Then I lifted my shirt and gave myself the shot.

Her eyes got wide and she asked, "Didn't that hurt?"

"Not at all" I said. "Do you think you can do it too?"

Hesitantly she agreed. With shaky hands, she drew up the saline, stuck the tiny needle into her tummy and pressed the plunger.

"Wow" she exclaimed, "that didn't hurt at all. I think I can do this!" She left with a follow-up appointment.

When I walked into the exam room two weeks later, there sat a very different Wanda. She looked up at me with a huge smile.

"Wait till you see my sugars!" she said. "I have been giving myself insulin every day and it is working! I can't thank you enough. Before you, nobody had ever taken the time to explain diabetes and its effect on me. You made all the difference!"

She got up and gave me a hug. In fact, her sugars had improved. She went from the 400s down to below 200 during the course of those two weeks. Her whole outlook on the disease had shifted.

Since then, I have watched Wanda modify her lifestyle. She has cut her A1C almost in half but more importantly, she is living her life. She does not have fear but has hope.

For me, when I think of Wanda and that first visit and where it has lead, I know that being a physician assistant is what I love. It is those very smiles and hugs I get when I am able to help that make everything I do worth the effort. They become the hooks that I grab onto when things get tough and challenging. They are WOW moments for me and are what keep me coming back for more!

Teri Pitman, PA-C, MSPAS
Endocrinology, San Diego

*"Caring about others, running the risk of feeling,
and leaving an impact on people,
brings happiness."*
Harold Kushner

It's Like She's Part of My Family

Ms. Hayes' father was a patient in the Observation Treatment Center at Kaiser Permanente Baldwin Park for three days. "The staff was excellent," she said but one particular nurse stood out, Glenna Reyes, RN.

The family had respected their father's wish not to be resuscitated. He had been ill for a long time and he and his family were accepting of the inevitable. There was usually someone from the family at the bedside both day and night. However, on the day he died, the family was not present.

When Ms. Hayes came back to the hospital she felt awful that she had not been there when her father passed away. Glenna came to her, expressed her sympathy and then sat down with her and described her father's last hours.

"As I sat and listened to Glenna, I couldn't stop staring at her and smiling inside," said Ms. Hayes. "I kept thinking 'it's like she's part of my family.' It meant so much to me to know that Glenna was there when we couldn't be. I felt such peace knowing that she was at my father's side during his last hours. Glenna is an angel."

In the words of one of Glenna's colleagues, "She is a beautiful example of the values and expectations of Kaiser Permanente. She represents her profession and this organization with the highest integrity. We are fortunate to have her as part of our team because her behavior on that day is typical of Glenna every day."

Glenna Reyes, RN was the recipient of a DAISY Award from Kaiser Permanente Baldwin Park.

Written and submitted by:
Yvonne Roddy-Sturm, RN
Clinical Director, Medical/Surgical/Critical Care, Baldwin Park

"Death leaves a heartache no one can heal,
love leaves a memory no one can steal."
From a headstone in Ireland

Will You Marry Me?

O ver the years working as a nurse, then later as a nurse practitioner, I have had the opportunity to meet some wonderful people. I have laughed and cried with them. I have watched their children grow, their parents die, and have held their hands through divorce and widowhood.

* * * * *

Early on as a new nurse practitioner I treated an elderly woman in her 80s. She had come in for her appointment with her daughter. She started telling me that her daughter had just turned 16 and about her husband at home who was, she said, 10 years her junior.

I decided to reorient her to the present. I gently and thoughtfully explained that her daughter was now in her 50s and that her late husband had passed away three years ago.

She looked at me, smiled, and simply replied, "Oh so that's where he's been!"

It was extremely difficult to keep a straight face. I just nodded my head and learned to leave well enough alone.

* * * * *

I was working as a case manager seeing patients in the hospital and after discharge, at their homes. I met Mr. Samuelson while he was hospitalized with congestive heart failure. He was 88 years old. After he was discharged, I spoke with him on the phone daily. He lived alone so I made a home visit to make sure that he was weighing himself and taking his medications properly. He would make trips to the office for follow-up visits with his doctor or with me.

About three months after his hospitalization, he came to the clinic to see me.

He was carrying a small box in his hand. He told me he had something very important he needed to discuss with me.

He sat down and gazed at me for a moment. He then proceeded to ask me to marry him and showed me the box holding the ring set that had belonged to his late wife. He explained that he wanted to marry me because his late wife and I shared the same name.

"It will be easy for me to remember your name once we are wed," he told me. He then showed me his checkbook to assure me that he had more than enough money to "take care of me." I smiled.

"I am so flattered by your proposal," I said not wanting to embarrass or hurt him in any way. "You are very kind and a good man but I am already married." He took it well and understood.

After he left, I started worrying about the bad things that could happen to him if he was carrying diamonds around and showing people his checkbook. I discussed it with his doctor. Finally, over the course of the next three months, I was able to persuade him to move into a retirement "villa."

It took a lot of convincing and in the end, the only way we could sway him was to tell him that a retirement villa would be the best place for him to meet a good woman. After his move, I heard he was the most sought after gentleman there!

Mary Hanson, FNP, MSN
Brea Medical Office, Orange County

*"Humor is the great thing, the saving thing. The minute it
crops up, all our irritations and resentments slip away
and a sunny spirit takes their place."*
Mark Twain

Thank You for Saving My Life

"Thank you for saving my life." Do you have any idea what it is like for a young nurse to hear those words? Hearing them reaffirmed why I chose nursing as my profession.

Mr. Roberts was a clinic patient admitted to the hospital for a number of problems. As a relatively new nurse, I had several patients that day including Mr. Roberts. I remember clearly that he was in a fully-occupied, four-bed room. He was at the far end of the room and distant from the nurse's station.

He was an older man who had worked for the Union Pacific Railroad for many years. Being in the hospital was difficult for him as it usually is for the patient, a time of uncertainty, discomfort and even fear.

That morning I was making my second patient round for the day shift. When I looked at Mr. Roberts, he seemed pale, diaphoretic and shaky.

"How are you feeling Mr. Roberts?" I asked him.

"I feel kind of funny," he replied.

"Funny? Can you describe it?" I asked. "Are you in pain?"

"No, I just feel funny," he said again.

I put on the call light. Someone came almost immediately. I asked for a sphygmomanometer and had one in my hands quickly.

In short order, I had taken his blood pressure and concerned with the results, started to call the doctor. Then realizing that this was a more urgent situation, I pulled the call light out of the wall and had everyone running down the hall to help. We were able to begin to reverse his symptoms, stabilize him and transfer him to ICU.

Several days later, Mr. Roberts was back in our unit and assigned to me again. The first thing he said when he saw me was "thank you for saving my life." He had vague memories of the incident but he said what he remembered was that I was calm and reassuring and how quickly I had gotten him the help he needed.

"I was in good hands," he said. "I knew everything would be all right."

Was I calm? No. Was I sure I was doing the right thing? No. But what counted was that he thought I had.

Even though I made an impact on him that day, he made an even bigger impact on me. Whether or not I actually saved his life doesn't matter. What mattered was that I was able to give him a sense of security, a sense of being cared for, and a sense of being safe when he needed those feelings the most.

It has been almost thirty years since that incident but I remember it as clear as yesterday. Those priceless words continue to reaffirm my choice of profession. The valuable lessons that I learned in those moments are a cornerstone in my work. I am proud to say that I am a nurse.

Joyce Johnson, RN-BC, PhD
SCPMG Regional Director, Education and Research, Pasadena

"People will forget what you said, people will forget what you did but people will never forget how you made them feel."
Maya Angelou

Little Hunches

"Hello, are you Judy?" the man asked me.

"Yes, I am," I answered.

The jolly gentleman standing in the lobby was rather robust and exuded kindness with his eyes and smile. He turned to the people sitting in the reception room and stated, "You are under great care. This lady has never met me, but she saved my life."

It happened not many days before. I had just opened a new Coumadin clinic in the Internal Medicine Department of the University of California, San Diego (UCSD). The list of individuals to call with INR results was rather large but I decided, as I always do, to start in on it one person at a time.

Mr. Raymond's name appeared and I noticed he was new to UCSD. I called him. It was a Friday. I left a message for him to call back. My sixth sense said he was not well so I called again before leaving for the upcoming Labor Day weekend. When I returned the following week, I immediately tried reaching Mr. Raymond and again there was no response.

For some reason, my internal radar was telling me to act without delay. I obtained his chart and called home health. I convinced them to go to his apartment because his information stated he lived alone.

Later in the afternoon, home health called saying they could not get into his apartment. I pressed on. I called the manager and had him open Mr. Raymond's apartment. Sure enough, he was found on his bed, unresponsive and barely breathing. He was rushed to the hospital where he remained on a ventilator for 12 days. Mr. Raymond was an undiagnosed COPD patient.

He told me later that if I had not listened to my inner thoughts, he would have died in his bed. I believe we all have our little hunches and they can prove to be helpful if you just listen to them.

Judy Gagne, RN
Urgent Appointment Clinic, San Diego

"Intuition is a spiritual faculty and does not explain, but simply points the way."
Florence Scovel Shinn

Star

My first job after graduating from nursing school was in a small New England town. It was the kind of place that could grace any Christmas issue magazine cover, including a town green complete with gazebo, little decorated trees and lots of snow.

The 85-bed hospital was just off this green. The hospital truly embraced the term community. We all lived, worked and played together in this small town. I often saw the outgoing charge nurse go through the entire floor and give a complete history of each patient to the oncoming shift without ever referring to the kardex. Even new patients were described in the kind of detail that would rival any biographical writer.

After awhile, I started seeing people who had been my patients. Family members of "frequent flyers" would come up to me and say thank you for something I had long forgotten; a pain medication given in time or a walk to the bathroom instead of using the commode that was the turning point in someone's recovery.

It was against this backdrop that Art came into my life. The first time I met him was in my nurse's aide days. He had had surgery and I took care of him during his recovery. I don't remember much about those encounters but Art remembered nearly all the details and recounted them to me when he came back into the hospital with oat cell carcinoma of the lungs.

By then, I was a graduate nurse on the Step Down Unit so my name badge read Elizabeth Spinella, GN. When Art saw it, he decided GN meant Great Nurse and took to calling me Star because I was a Great Nurse. I tried correcting him, but he wouldn't hear of it. So, I was Star.

All patients receiving chemotherapy came to my unit. At the time, in 1980, chemotherapy consisted primarily of Cisplantinium drips run over two to three days with lots of vomiting and hair loss. As a graduate nurse, I could not "hang chemo," but I could take care of the patients.

I worked a split shift, three nights and two days each week. It made for a crazy lifestyle, but it meant I saw my oncology patients during the day when life was hopeful and at night when life frequently got scary. Over time I came to appreciate this dynamic. My patients taught me a great deal about life and death.

The next time Art came in for another round of chemotherapy, he spotted me immediately, said hello and asked me if I was his nurse again. After report, I requested Art as my patient. I remembered him as a fun-loving, easygoing kind of person.

I knew he had a terrible cancer, but he seemed so upbeat. I was hopeful for him. Art was assigned to me as a return patient whenever I was working.

The first few rounds of chemotherapy went considerably well for Art. His positive attitude was his biggest shield to the side effects. His support system of friends and family all helped. In fact, he started a game with me called "find the empty beer cans."

Yes, Art's friends would sneak in beer and after I would discharge him from the hospital, I would find beer cans hidden in different locations around the room. Upon his next admission, he would ask me if I had found all of them.

The first time it happened, his little game shook me up and I grew concerned for his safety. I reported it immediately to my charge nurse. But over time, and as his condition worsened, for better or worse, I just let it go.

During the day, Art was the happy-go-lucky person that everyone knew, but my heart was touched the most at night. I would bring him his liquid morphine, a blue solution in a medicine cup. He would drink it down and then I would sit with him as he looked out the window and talked about life and the wisdom that impending death brings.

I wish I could remember all that he said, but I can't. I just remember listening to him, sometimes feeling over my head, sometimes not feeling very much like a Star.

But I can still see him sitting in the bed leaning on the over-the-bed table, quietly waiting for me to return.

Art didn't die on my shift. I don't think he wanted me to do the postmortem care. I had had other patients die, but he was the first one that truly hit my heart. I cannot say I was sad. I was actually relieved but then again I was only 22 years old. Art was my first true connection with death.

Liz Spinella-Jones, RN, MPA
Department Administrator, Internal Medicine, Rheumatology and
Infectious Diseases, Woodland Hills

*"A bit of fragrance always clings to
the hand that gives roses."*
Chinese Proverb

Who Knew!

As nurse-midwives, we may never know the impact we have on someone's life. In the hectic, occasionally mundane days of a large office and hospital practice, we often take for granted the unique care we, as midwives, provide. In my 35 years of midwifery practice, three special women reminded me of how a short encounter can change a life.

The first was a woman who had a routine normal delivery. I met her and her family that day and we shared a few hours of labor and the miracle of her baby's birth. Nothing stood out in my mind as atypical or extraordinary and I soon forgot the delivery. Eight years later, I received an unexpected letter from her.

She wrote about the day that she gave birth as the most wonderful, memorable day of her life primarily due to my encouraging her to help deliver her infant and place him on her abdomen. She looked back on that time and the sense of empowerment she experienced, and felt the need eight years afterward to let me know. Who knew!

A few years later, I received another unexpected letter from a woman who recently delivered her first child. I had met her two or three years earlier during a prior pregnancy that did not result in a live birth. At that time, during her initial OB visit, we discussed many issues, including her risk as a Caucasian of carrying a recessive gene for cystic fibrosis.

Initially, she chose not to be tested but changed her mind after further discussion. Indeed, she was a carrier and was very angry with me for supporting testing and making her needlessly worry. Unfortunately, her husband was also a carrier, affecting the fetus.

She faced a very difficult decision and a very traumatic period in her life. Her guilt and grief were profound. But years later, as she recounted her many untold emotions toward me, she thanked me for the time I took to discuss the testing with her and how it changed the future of her family. Who knew!

The final patient involved a woman with a body mass index in the grossly obese category. I saw her for a routine annual exam and we discussed her future fertility plans. She already had some menstrual issues and her weight placed her at risk for infertility and adverse pregnancy outcomes. We had a lengthy discussion regarding food choices and exercise.

She left annoyed that I overtly addressed her weight and health risks. However, she thought about our conversation and decided to change her life because two years later, she was back in my office unrecognizable and 150 pounds thinner.

She openly wept as she related her feelings of power and confidence. She felt ready to face parenthood. Although other providers told her she was fat, no one had taken time to discuss the specifics of changing her lifestyle. Who knew!

As nurse-midwives, we connect with women on very intimate and personal levels and we empower women to manage their health. I am grateful to these three women who took the time to let me know how each brief encounter impacted their futures. They reminded me that, even though we may never know, each visit is important to the women we serve.

Sue Nadig-Wall, CNM, MSN
Retired, Orange County

"When we do the best we can, we never know
what miracle is wrought in our life,
or in the life of another."
Helen Keller

In Control

The spiritual lady from Los Angeles was retired. She regularly cared for her grandchildren after school, had completed the family reunion, laughed often with her daughter and was preparing her garden for springtime, when suddenly she was stricken with slurred speech and a headache.

These symptoms had been occurring over a few days when her daughter intuitively stopped by from work only to find her mother overcome with the classic signs of a stroke. She scooped her up and took her to urgent care.

The CAT scan showed a mass. The physician told the daughter that her mother required admission to the hospital because she needed further tests. The diagnosis—glioblastoma—came as a shock. The tumor was incapacitating her quickly and removing it was the only choice.

During surgery, the biopsy confirmed the malignancy. The spiritual lady opted for no radiation and no chemotherapy. She recovered from the brain surgery with few complications and her daughter took her home about 10 days later. The discharge plan included hospice, because of her wishes for no further treatment.

When we met the spiritual lady and her daughter, we saw a very alert woman. The incision on her scalp had almost healed and her beautiful gray hair had nearly grown back from the surgical shaving.

As we carefully explained our hospice services, it became very apparent that this patient and her family wanted to stay in complete control. The daughter told us that her mother was on a six-week raw food diet, that herbs were her preferred choice of medicinal therapy, and that she walked around the block on a daily basis. The patient told us "that her spirit was with the Lord, that his guidance was her way."

Her demeanor, considering such a devastating diagnosis and prognosis, impressed us. Actually, the patient and her family uplifted us as we completed our paperwork for admission to our program.

Back at the office, we discussed the situation. The family's desire for independence was purely positive but we knew we had to gain their trust. Seizure activity, falling, anxiety and the potential for pain would likely arise because of the patient's prognosis. We needed to pave the way for our future recommendations to assist with these symptoms as they occurred.

The team, inclusive of the physician, the nurse and the social worker, met with the family. We set up a short-term strategy to order some durable medical equipment in the home for safety and to introduce medications that would assist with potential symptoms.

The spiritual lady made it through her raw food diet and celebrated her birthday by eating her favorite cake but began to require assistance with her activities of daily living. She used more equipment, could not shower any longer, nor take her walks due to weakness of her legs, her arms and the drooping of her face. Although these changes were difficult for the family to watch, we felt their spirit and faith with each visit we made.

The trust with the hospice team and the caregiver daughter grew stronger as the patient became more bed bound. The mother eventually required 24-hour care. The daughter and her family moved in to share her remaining time. It was truly about the quality of days. They knew in their hearts that it was not about the quantity. Their church family became an added, constant source of support.

This patient and family gave the hospice team such inspiration. The daughter always greeted us with a great big smile and the gospel music in the background reminded us of the faith that the spiritual lady shared with us on the day we became part of her life.

Providing hospice care for patients and families facing death is difficult and yet rewarding at the same time. This patient and family gave us the memories of a rewarding experience at such a critical moment in the circle of life.

Teresa Mountain, RN

Director, Patient Care Services, Hospice/Palliative Care Programs, Los Angeles

"Because I have loved life,
I shall have no sorrow to die."

Amelia Burr

No Ordinary
Hospital Shower

This story is about a patient who impacted an entire department and how that entire department "payed it forward" by impacting her with their unique gifts of time, compassion and friendship.

Dee Dee was a 24-year-old, first-time mom-to-be, expecting twins. A pregnancy-related problem kept her confined to the hospital. The staff described her as calm, polite, cooperative and a person who put the welfare of her babies ahead of her own personal needs.

Dee Dee clearly knew that she needed continual monitoring. She took quick showers so that she could return to bed to have her babies back on the monitor as soon as possible. She let the nurses know when she was getting up so they wouldn't worry that her tracing was not recording. She was self-reliant and learned how to plug and unplug her monitor so that she maintained her independence whenever possible.

She chose to dress every day and change into her pajamas each evening as though she were at home. She created a personal space in her hospital room with personal pictures and mementos from her college alma mater, the University of Southern California (USC).

At times, she would study for the LSAT, her goal being to become a lawyer. She would wear a USC sweatshirt while enjoying movies on her laptop. She was inspiring, never losing sight of her goal for healthy babies and her dream of becoming a lawyer.

The entire staff recognized Dee Dee's outstanding qualities and admired her ability to remain herself. She never allowed her circumstances to dictate how she "showed up" for her day. Everyone realized that this stay in the hospital ruled out the possibility of her experiencing what most new moms-to-be get to enjoy, a baby shower to celebrate the upcoming birth of her treasured babies.

The nurses in Labor and Delivery decided to host a surprise baby shower for Dee Dee and her spouse. They provided food and a cake along with gifts and words of encouragement, creating a wonderful memory for her and supporting her in a very special way. The family was overwhelmed with emotion at the outpouring of compassion and caring that these nurses "showered" on them.

When we take time to care, to see and to experience the life of others, beautiful things can happen. This memory left an indelible mark, not only on this patient, but also on the hearts of those nurses who cared enough to make a difference in the lives of their patients.

Written and submitted on behalf of the Labor and Delivery staff nurses by:
Lynda Mayer, RN, MHA
Director, Maternal-Child Health, Los Angeles

"Happiness cannot come from without. It must come from within. It is not what we see and touch or that which others do for us which makes us happy; it is that which we think and feel and do, first for the other fellow and then for ourselves."
Helen Keller

Crushed Skull

Such a beautiful day
What could possibly go wrong?

Hmmm, flashing lights on the freeway
Only police with bodies on the ground
Should I stop?

A physician, I say
Are you sure? he said
ID cleared the air

Such a peaceful scene
Mom and dad as if asleep on the front seat
I knew better

A small child, on the back seat lay still
It was "just a rear-ender," I thought
Precious memories of my own loved ones, flooded my mind

Funny, not a bit of blood to be seen anywhere
A touch to his small skull made it clear
His life would soon be over

I wonder when I'll stop feeling, the crushed skull, probably never…

One Sunday morning about six months ago, I was driving back from seeing an old friend in Los Angeles. At the junction of the 605 and the 105, the traffic was jammed. I could see ahead that there was an accident. As I approached, I saw only CHP cars and bodies on the ground.

I have learned over the years that doctors who show up at a medical emergency when medics are on the scene are not always welcomed. The medics can do just about everything I can in a field situation. But this was a different circumstance so I stopped.

It was chaotic. The officer on the scene intercepted me. I identified myself as an emergency physician. He asked for my identification, which I produced. "This guy says he's a doc," he announced to his partner.

I went to the car with the most damage ready to use the Hoag triage method "START" but it was clear at first glance that the two adults in the front seat were not going to "stand up and move over here." Some CHP officers were maintaining their airways.

It appeared as though a van had rear-ended the car at what must have been a very high rate of speed. So much so that the rear seat back was at a 45-degree angle from the right rear to the back of the driver side seat. The child in the back seemed to have been sitting on a booster seat with a belt, but the impact of the crash had violently launched him.

On the seat lay an unconscious four- to five-year old male. Essentially, there was no blood in sight on the child. He had sonorous breathing. I carefully opened his airway and maintained c-spine inline traction. His breathing improved. That was when I felt what seemed like a broken eggshell inside of a thick plastic bag. He remained totally non-responsive.

The medics finally arrived after what seemed like an eternity. The first medic on the scene ordered me to let go of the child and back out of the car. I identified myself as a physician and respectfully refused saying, "I'm not going to let go of his c-spine."

Soon, another appeared with a stabilization device and I backed out. I heard one medic say to the other that the child's pulse was 80. I think by this time the child was getting close to herniation.

There was nothing more for me to do, so I continued on my way. Concerned about the head injury of this child, I called the local trauma center on a hunch that a critical trauma child might wind up there.

I spoke with one of the nurses who said that a critical trauma was on the way. I suggested that they might want to call in a pediatric neurosurgeon. She was very thankful that I had called.

I called back a few days later and found out the child was brain dead and on life support. His skull indeed crushed like an eggshell. I spoke with the trauma coordinator nurse about a potential educational opportunity for the medics-on-scene thinking to perhaps increase awareness of head traumas. She was receptive.

The whole thing stayed with me for awhile maybe because of being outside the imaginary security of an ER. I had one of those sentient moments after writing this short poem when I realized I could relax a bit.

Richard Pitts, DO
Occupational Medicine and Emergency Medicine, Orange County

"Knowledge is learning something every day.
Wisdom is letting go of something every day."
Zen Proverb

The Benefits of Exercise

I had worked at Kaiser Permanente as a diabetes educator for about a year, when I met him for the first time. He had just buried his wife and partner of 60 years. With the utmost sympathy, I told him that I could not even comprehend what that would feel like, the loss, the permanent separation with no hope of retrieval.

My background had included working with very depressed patients and, at the time, I was working on a Master of Nursing in Psychiatric/Mental Health. I had firsthand experience seeing improvement with depressed patients if we could get them walking. For this man, it would be walking off his grief. So, I encouraged him to start at a gentle pace either walking or riding a stationary bike with specific instructions not to exceed his exertion tolerance.

I didn't see him for almost a year. When he returned to my office for a visit, he looked great. He cupped his hands around his mouth as he whispered to me, "I have a secret. Can I tell you?"

"Of course," I said encouraging him to share with me, thinking he was going to tell me that perhaps he had a new partner.

"I'm having sex," he whispered with great secrecy. "I thought that was over years ago. I wish I'd known about this exercise thing sooner. I knew exercise was a big 'to do' for lowering blood glucose, but wow, I never realized that it would help my sex life.

"You need to tell all your patients about the great benefits that exercise can bring," he said. "Here I am, an 85-year-old man, re-enjoying what I thought was gone many years ago. I have to thank you for getting me to do it."

He was effervescent. He told me that he had started slowly, but gradually, he was able to do more. The more he did, the better he felt. I wondered whether he was talking about sex or exercise but then he told me he had worked up to walking about five miles daily or rode his stationary bike about 10 miles daily.

I was amazed but did not ask for more information fearing other details he might tell me. As I ushered him out I said, "Keep up the good work" realizing too late the possible double meaning.

"Thank you again," he replied with a twinkle in his eye. "My 'work' is really doing great. Yes indeedeee."

Marlyn "Marli" Crane, RN
Diabetes Case Manager, Preventive Medicine, Fontana

"The only thing that should surprise us is that there are still some things that can surprise us."
Francois De La Rochefoucauld

Thoughts from Perioperative Nurses to New Graduates

While there are many books available to describe the mechanics of being an operating room nurse, to my knowledge, there has been nothing written to describe what it is really like.

"Operating room nursing is many things, always different, always changing."

"You need to be innovative at times, and to have some mechanical ability as well."

"It is fast paced, but sometimes, in the middle of a really long procedure, time can seem to stubbornly stand still. You can almost visualize the healing process beginning before your eyes, and wonder if you have missed celebrating any birthdays."

"You certainly must enjoy working as a team, but realize that there is no captain of this ship; you are all working together! The captain does not keep the ship afloat. Even the Titanic sank under the leadership of a great captain. External factors affect our 'ship' every day."

"Realize that nearly everyone in the operating room is a 'Type A' personality. Don't eat your young. Teach others in a way that you were taught or wish you had been taught."

"There is nothing more rewarding than the successful completion of a difficult procedure either due to the surgery itself, to the medical condition of your patient, or to your contribution as an operating room nurse."

"I'm glad you're considering the operating room as your career choice. I'm sure you've found a few people who have said 'yuck that's not real nursing.' It IS real nursing, but can be hard to describe to someone whose frame of reference is medical-surgical nursing, coronary care nursing or rehabilitation nursing."

"Bear in mind that there are few places where a patient is so totally reliant on his or her nurse than when they are having surgery. The nurse needs to consider everything from the patient's skin and subcutaneous tissue health to their organ function, from their family dynamics to their electrolyte balance, from their prior surgical history to their wishes for end-of-life treatment, from their range of motion to their allergies, plus, a few more."

"Operating room nurses have such a limited time to make a difference. Gone are the days when the nurse can do a leisurely pre-op visit the evening before surgery, chatting with the patient and his or her family about what will happen the next day. Our focus now has to be to get the right information, plan and implement the appropriate care based on that information, and make the correct adjustments as they occur."

"Operating room nurses must be good at thinking outside the box. Every patient follows a different path, even though they may be having the same procedure as their neighbor. The nurse who can consider all usual solutions to a problem and can come up with several new options has the best chance of succeeding in a typical operating room."

"I love the operating room! I am glad that I have the opportunity to work there, and I would choose it all over again if I were a new graduate."

Collected by:
Marie H. Paulson, RN, BSN, MS, CNOR
Manager, Perioperative Practice Specialist, Pasadena

"There's a difference between interest and commitment. When you're interested in doing something, you do it only when it's convenient. When you're committed to something, you accept no excuses; only results."
Kenneth Blanchard

Ryan the Lion

Coming back from vacation is always difficult and when I came back in mid-June after two weeks off, the unit seemed especially busy. On my second day back, I approached one of our longtime NICU nurses to talk with her. Screens were around the bedside, possibly a bad sign. I knew this baby to be a 2-week-old, very tiny baby. Cathy, the nurse, explained to me that a care conference had just finished, and that the doctor had given the parents the option of discontinuing life support.

Just as she finished this statement, the baby's dad came over to Cathy and indicated they had decided to proceed with cessation later that day, and that he and his wife didn't think they could be present. Without missing a beat, Cathy said "well, then I will hold him for you." Cathy had just returned to work after losing her husband to a difficult battle with cancer. Her offer brought tears to my eyes.

Cathy and her peers helped these young parents hold their baby, and take many pictures with the many family members who were present, the only pictures Ryan would ever be part of. Cathy helped them bathe and diaper their baby for the first time, and rub lotion over his tiny body. Pictures of a tiny face with no tape (tube removed), last kisses, lots of tears, gifts of patience and tender care given, and moments shared made a long bittersweet good-bye.

Ryan was 26-weeks gestation, and weighed only 650 grams. His parents had waited for him for a long time. He was their first baby. His course in our NICU was stormy and not uncommon for his gestation. He was with us only 16 days. Now, nearly every memory his parents have of him will forever be involved with NICU. Did we do everything we could for this baby and his parents?

My answer came several days later when Betsy, another seasoned NICU nurse came to me with tales of Ryan's funeral. It was at that time I realized the NICU staff had given so much more than just a sweet good-bye.

One of our NICU nurses, Vicki, a 30-year veteran, draws simple cartoon animal pictures with colored pencils, then carefully letters the baby's name and hangs them at the bedside, in prominent view. Vicki drew a picture of a lion for Ryan. He quickly became Ryan the Lion.

This theme carried through his funeral, with the decorations being stuffed lions. His mother spoke about his spirit at his service, referring to Ryan the Lion. His head stone bears a lion that looks remarkably like the one Vicki drew, and under his name, Ryan the Lion. We helped his parents learn about his character and see his strength.

It is a common practice for nurses to encourage parents to bring pictures to put into their little one's isolette. Having no other children, Ryan's parents brought pictures of their pets at home. Jennifer added dialogue bubbles, indicating that these pets were anxiously waiting to meet this new little baby. She also wrote a card to mom and dad from Ryan when he was a week old, talking about how much stronger he had gotten. Mom and dad received these items along with a photograph of Ryan. They were on display at the funeral, now each a prized possession and a happy memory.

During the eulogy, Ryan's parents acknowledged multiple NICU staff for their contributions not only to their son's care but for the support given to them. Ryan had surgery three days before he died. His parents were desperately worried. Sandy, Ryan's nurse, came to the waiting room every 15 minutes during the surgery, updating them on his progress. Her support and constant flow of information really helped them to cope.

Betsy gave Ryan wonderful baby massages along with answers to any questions his parents asked. Shelia listened and helped them realize that there probably wasn't a miracle in store for their baby. She reassured them that he wasn't in pain. And the list went on.

Ryan died on June 16, 2008, held by his dad, with his mom right beside. It was at shift change. Many of his nurses were there and cried with his parents.

People tell me frequently that they could not do my job. My answer to each of them is the same. I can do my job because I work with incredible people who care deeply about what they do, and they do it well in the worst of circumstances.

Annette Adams, RN, MSN
Department Administrator, NICU, Fontana

"We can do no great things, only small things with great love."
Mother Teresa

More Than a
Stamp Collection

When asked to write about a moving experience in my chosen career, ideas did not come as easily as I thought they would. Given more than a decade of nursing, I should have a treasure trove of stories. I believe in the deep recesses of my mind that I do, although I would have to sit down and give them time to rise to the surface. But, for now, instead of story after story, what came to me are a myriad of memories that formed the small wonders that touched not only me, but the souls who surrounded those days.

A wheelchair ride, a terminally ill 17-year-old's last wish, before he succumbed to leukemia a day after we took that final trip along the unit's hallway.

A mother's wish to hold her child an extra hour after the baby's death.

A football team dedicates their winning game to their fallen teammate, while he lay in his hospital bed battling the debilitating effects of chemotherapeutic drugs.

A charitable foundation formed after a family's ordeal with a rare chronic neuro-muscular disease affecting their infant son. He was just 5 months old; the medical team thought reaching the age of 1 would be shooting for the moon. Now 3, he and his family continue to inspire us, turning what was once an unfortunate situation into one that could possibly bring hope to future victims of such a rarity. The foundation intends to aid impoverished children from the family's native country.

A few baptisms, we nurses, as healers, have partaken as the newborn earth angels transcend to angels in heaven.

Our hands have held the children's hands allowing them to squeeze hard hoping to alleviate the pain that comes with needle sticks and procedures.

We have held the hands of families facing the harsh reality that their loved one would not make it to see the sunrise. When the room fills with such silence and random sobs echo that not a word can be said, we, nurses, were there in those darkest moments.

We are living witnesses to many firsts and lasts. We were there to hear a newborn's first cry, first breath and first vaccine. We have aided a child's first hours of recovery from a surgical procedure, the last day for a leg cast and the first day to walk without crutches. We have seen the last day for someone's heart and liver but a first and new beginning for someone else in dire need of new ones. We have beheld the first blessing of the sick and the anointing before their last breath.

While some may have a collection of antiques, treasured heirlooms, stamps or vintage cars, we, nurses, have this rare collection of days in the lives of people we have encountered. From the outside looking in, we can see our image as a mother, a sister, a friend, a messenger, an aide, a ray of hope, a bridge between two lives, the coming and the passing, and most of all as a healer. Through stages of life, there was and will always be a spot where we stand and, with or without knowing, we have filled a space that made a difference in the lives of others.

Aileen Oswald, RN
Pediatric Intensive Care Unit, Los Angeles

"What we have done for ourselves alone dies with us. What we have done for others and the world remains and is immortal."
Albert Pine

The Wrong Connection

I remember vividly sitting on that cold stainless steel stool at the head of the OR bed staring into the face of a woman about to have eye surgery. I was a student nurse anesthetist, with three months training under my belt, about to give this woman a general anesthetic for her delicate operation.

My clinical instructor walked in and stood against the back wall leaving me to push all the drugs through the IV line. Peter, my classmate, and I had worked on a one-of-a-kind system of stopcocks inserted between the IV tubing and the extension line going to the patient. Here I would inject my IV anesthesia drugs, and smoothly and atraumatically induce sleep; thus impressing all in the room.

However, this plan took a slight wrong turn. With everything and everyone in place, I pushed the 20 ml syringe and lo and behold the liquid squirted into my ear! What a cold shock this was to me! Trying quickly to assess what went wrong, I decided this was not the time or place to trace the pathway to the patient. So, I took the syringe and put a needle onto it and planned to use the rubber cap in the tubing to inject my drugs—Plan B.

Shaky and embarrassed, I turned to inject the rubber cap and nicked my thumb hard enough to start a stream of my blood splattering everywhere, visible to all! Where was my guardian angel now? I needed HELP! With a deep breath and the use of gauze and tape, I restored my composure and control of the situation. But, now I had to get my grade. How much worse could this situation get?

My instructor, John Garde, was ready for me at the end of the day with my case summation. "Your didactic scoring was satisfactory, however, your clinical skills need polishing up," he said. "Next time, connect the stopcock to the IV line not to the precordial stethoscope line running to your earpiece."

With that bit of wisdom, I hurriedly tried to escape the room when I heard his voice say, "Today was a good start in your anesthesia career. You'll be alright!" Thank God for wise instructors who are awesome people!

Rosanne Padovich, CRNA

Assistant Department Administrator, Anesthesia, Los Angeles

"Thorns and stings
And those such things
Just make stronger
Our angel wings."
Emme Woodhull-Bäche

Emotional Sutures

Helping a client heal on a deeper emotional level is pivotal to a client healing on the physical level. At least that is my belief. The more traumatic the incident, the more the spiritual and emotional aspect needs to be addressed.

One morning I received an intake call from a plastic surgeon to assist a 24-year-old female patient. She had been living with a mentally ill sister who had a long history of paranoid schizophrenia. They didn't get along.

Her sister was often off her medications and would hallucinate badly. In one such episode, she thought the patient was the devil. In a delusional tirade, the sister stabbed the patient about 18 times.

The patient was taken to the University of California, Los Angeles (UCLA) Medical Center where she was sutured and stabilized, but she needed a further consultation about surgery on her thumb. As a Kaiser Permanente member, her follow-up needed to be at a Kaiser Permanente facility, in this case, the West Los Angeles (WLA) Medical Center. UCLA stated the surgery was urgent and advised her to go through the ER.

Coming into the ER is hard for anyone because the environment tends to be intense, chaotic, fast and sometimes impersonal. Imagine coming into the hospital with multiple stab wounds on your face, hands and body, after just being released from another facility.

When the patient arrived, no one knew what was needed because her records were still at UCLA. The plastic surgeon wanted me to assist in coordinating her care. Her primary care physician was in Bellflower, another Kaiser Permanente facility, but the surgeon was in WLA.

The patient was surprisingly calm and collected when she discussed her experience.

One of her biggest fears was returning to the home she shared with her sister. Additionally, her mother wasn't supportive because she was both in denial and embarrassed by the assault within the family. The patient felt alone and victimized. I knew she needed emotional sutures.

I engaged her and offered supportive listening. I told her I would get her through the system. I knew any struggle to get treatment and services would feel to her like another assault.

First, I assisted her in finding a new place to live for both her safety as well as her physical and emotional healing. I connected her to Victims of Violent Crime; they helped with relocation expenses. Luckily, her sister was incarcerated which bought some time.

Next, I connected with her physician in Bellflower, who was very responsive and authorized treatment. I called member services about her medical records from UCLA. They were right there to coordinate care.

I helped her gain more support in her personal life. The patient already had a wonderful minister who was supportive and provided a spiritual understanding for her wounded, betrayed and deeply hurt soul. I contacted psychiatry to assist her in attending therapy to work on the emotional trauma resulting from the family violence.

Every time I connected her to a resource and received a result, I felt like I was stitching up her emotional body. Every resource became a suture, helping her to feel heard and giving her the energetic empathy her family could not provide.

Lessening the enormity of trying to gain services in a large health care organization, where it is easy to feel lost, was another stitch. Assisting the patient in feeling a personal connection to someone in the organization who was a supporter and an advocate was another suture.

As a psychotherapist, I believed if the client was emotionally cared for and her spirit supported, her physical healing would surely follow. The mind, body and spirit are intertwined.

The patient was very strong and confident about 'testifying' about her experience in church and was positive she would heal. Someone attempted to stab her to death, but she was somehow stabbed to life, finding more of a purpose and reason for her tragedy.

I admired her courage and felt satisfied that I provided her with a healing experience, if only through a couple of phone calls.

The last time I talked to the patient was on August 28, 2007. On August 29, 2008, almost exactly a year to date since I last made contact, I called her to see how she was doing and ask her permission to tell her story.

Synchronicities always mean something. She was thrilled to hear about her story being told. She has moved out-of-state and has restarted her life. Her plans are to start law school and ultimately practice family law. She remembered me.

"I still have your voicemail message on my cell phone," she said. "I've had it for a year because I wanted to follow-up with you." I was stunned that she would save my message for so long but I guess my voice was a healing balm, a positive memory during a nightmare.

My intention was to give her support and empathy during the worst trauma of her life. She validated that the services I had provided were a set of emotional sutures and she still had not removed that one last stitch.

Carolyn Coleridge, MSW
Social Medicine, West Los Angeles

"*No act of kindness, however small, is ever wasted.*"
Aesop

Kindness Can
Work Wonders

Before my surgery, I did everything possible to ensure the best outcome— researched my condition, secured a highly recommended surgeon, met with the anesthesiologist, updated my durable power of attorney and invested in some new pajamas. If you're going to be recuperating for up to six weeks, you want to do it in style.

On my last day of work before surgery, I watched in horror as planes exploded into the World Trade Center. Would Los Angeles be next? Might it happen during or after my surgery? How much stress was now added to an already stressful hospital work environment?

Arriving at Kaiser Permanente Los Angeles in the wee hours of the morning, I hugged my anxious husband and my worried parents goodbye. My innermost thoughts, "I want my dog, my couch and a big dish of ice cream."

Resigned to be an adult, I put on my goofy cap and gown, shoved my belongings into a plastic bag and began dreading the IV, since my "submarine" veins always present an uncomfortable challenge. Instructions from medical personnel were going in one ear and out the other.

As they wheeled my gurney toward the OR, a head wearing my same silly cap popped into view and said, "Well, if it isn't Lisa Beezley."

"Huh?" I mumbled.

"I'm Marilyn. You may not remember me, but I've seen you act in almost every play you've been in at the Colony Theatre," she said.

"I'm your recovery nurse," Marilyn continued. "I'll be the first person you see when you wake up. If you're experiencing any pain, just let me know, and I'll take care of it."

Wow! Everything changed for me in that one magical moment. Did I remember Marilyn? Of course I did! Suddenly I felt myself relax. My confidence grew three sizes.

I thanked her for the reassurance as she disappeared down the hall. Once inside the operating room, my heroine surgeon appeared.

"Are you ready to do this?" she asked. I said yes, but now I meant it.

Later, I awoke in recovery to a great deal of pain. Although Marilyn appeared blurry, there she was, ready to take care of me. My guardian angel, I thought.

Now, whenever I see Marilyn at the theatre, I introduce her just that way, as my guardian angel. "It was nothing," she always replies blushingly, "just part of my job." But I tell her each time that her reassurance meant so much to me.

Moving ever closer to the operating room, you'd be hard-pressed to find a human being who doesn't feel vulnerable and scared. Often, just a few kind words can make all the difference. In fact, they can work wonders.

Lisa Beezley-Lippman
CareActors Manager, Educational Theatre Programs Department, Pasadena

"Unless someone like you cares a whole awful lot,
nothing is going to get better. It's not."
Dr. Seuss

So Many Names
So Many Faces

So many names
So many faces
All races
All ages
Breast cancer respects no one
How can we end this disease?
Only through research

The journey begins
From Santa Barbara to Malibu
Three days of walking
Sleeping on the ground in tents
Port-a-potties and port-a-showers
Sharing stories
Sharing caring for a disease that touches so many lives

Walkers for grandmothers, wives, mothers, daughters, sisters, aunts and friends
I walk to honor memories
For all of my patients on this journey called breast cancer
For a friend/coworker who barely made her 40th birthday
For a wonderful Breast Buddy volunteer who could never have enough
    "Buddies" to help
For a young mother with children so small they would have no real memories
    of their mom

I had trained, prepared, even used exercise poles
My mantra as I walked was "I hate breast cancer"
Each day along the route, there were many spectators
Cheering, words of encouragement, clapping, whistling, waving signs
Check points for water or juice or Gatorade and a small snack
So many wonderful volunteers

The last day proved the hardest
The Santa Monica Mountains along Highway 1
Hot, very hot
A checkpoint with big squirt guns helped cool us down
"Keep going, you can do it," I say to a young woman in tears walking for
        her sister

In the end, I raised over $4000
But something was wrong
In my mind, the walk had not been difficult enough
An inadequate gesture to honor the strong, brave, resilient, kind, generous,
        loving women that I have watched on their journey of breast cancer
I had to find something else

I have always hated tattoos
It would be very difficult for me to do
A breast cancer ribbon with a rose through the loop in memory of those lost
A butterfly perched for those who survive
Around my left ankle for the entire world to see
My commitment to the women who battle this disease every day

We must not forget
So many names
So many faces
Each one an important life
Each woman and her family that have crossed my path have left their mark
      on me
Forever

These amazing women
My life changed for the better
I look forward to coming to work
Who will I meet next?
How will I help them through their journey?

Laura L. Ward, RN, CPSN, OCN
Breast Care Coordinator, Plastic Surgery, Fontana

Hook, Line and Sinker

My nursing career changed in 1994. After having worked as an LVN for 20 years, mostly in orthopedics and primary care, a reduction in workforce brought me to the Hematology/Oncology Department. I had planned to keep the position for a short time while looking for something else, but the people who work in this field and the patients we care for captured my soul.

It started slowly at first, the urge to lay a hand on someone's shoulder, a patient's family asking me to pray with them or someone that I helped get through a difficult biopsy who said "thank you." I was in it for the long run, grabbed as the saying goes—hook, line and sinker. I had found my place in an area that might not be the most popular, but is so rewarding that every day I can be at peace knowing this is where I make a difference.

The first patient I became close to was a female Christian marriage counselor. She was 82-years young, still practicing her faith and her counseling. She arranged her chemotherapy sessions around her clients. This beautiful vivacious woman never doubted where she was going. She understood the severity of her disease and yet she arrived with a smile and a gentle touch for everyone she met.

Through her, I learned that cancer can be like any other ailment. Fighting is the way through, but living is the answer. She lived to be 94. When she died, I was sad that I would never have long conversations with her again and yet knew she helped me to help others with wisdom and love.

I treat each patient with an understanding of how precious life is; meeting their families and becoming attached is part of being, just as death fulfills the circle of life. I mourn the loss, celebrate the victories, and choose to be part of the extended family of patients and coworkers that make up this team. My duty to nursing is a joy and a gift that I am thankful for at the end of each day. I believe that when we make a difference in someone's life, they in turn make a difference in ours.

Suzanne Shumate, LVN
LVN Team Leader, Hematology/Oncology, Orange County

"I am a part of all that I have met."
Alfred, Lord Tennyson

Nursing is in the
Miracle Moments

As an NICU nurse for over 28 years, I have countless precious memories of past patients and their families. Nursing a tiny premature baby or a sick newborn for weeks and often months, allows one to develop a unique and special bond. Supporting parents through such stressful times and watching them move from terrified, helpless "deer-in-the-headlights" new parents, to confident and competent caretakers, is perhaps the ultimate reward. These relationships grow, strengthened by sharing and deepening trust, and thus are ripe with tender insights, personal struggles and quiet triumphs. I call them Miracle Moments.

One morning, as I entered the nurse's station, I found out that we had a special new admit. Baby Jason had been born with amniotic band injuries to his limbs. His right leg had been amputated below the knee in utero, and he had been born with a tight band around his right arm that had severely diminished the blood supply to his lower arm and hand. He required emergency surgery the night before to remove the band. His family was quite distraught and struggling to cope with this unexpected problem.

I was eager to take this baby because I wanted to comfort his family by sharing the story of my brother. He, too, had been born with a below-the-elbow amputation and it had not held him back a bit. I imagined talking to them about his career in the dive industry as an instructor and underwater photographer. I wanted to provide encouragement by assuring them of his completely non-handicapped life.

I approached the family near the baby's isolette and introduced myself. When I asked gently how they were doing, they completely surprised me by turning around and beaming at me!

"We're doing GREAT," his mother said.

"Wow! Tell me about it." I said.

They went on to share that they had been in agony the night before because they had to sign a surgical consent that included the words "...and possible amputation of lower right arm and hand."

"We could imagine life without a leg," his mother said.

"A prosthesis is no big deal. It can be hidden underneath pants," said his dad.

They thought they could cope with that reality. But they could not imagine life for a boy, and later a man, without his hand. How would he do all the things that boys and men need to do?

Throughout the surgery, they had paced and prayed with their extended family in the lobby of the hospital on the first floor. Suddenly, right before their eyes walked a man missing his right arm below the elbow! He was well-dressed, seemingly relaxed and happy, and accompanied by his pregnant wife.

"Our jaws dropped and we just stared after him all the way down the hall," the mother said.

"We realized that God had just answered our prayers and sent us proof, in the flesh, that a man with one arm could be successful and confident," said the dad.

The man they saw was obviously able to attract a beautiful wife, have a family and lead what looked like a completely normal life. They had wept with relief and intuitively knew that in spite of the obstacles, their son would be okay.

I was beaming by now. There was no need to share with them the story of my brother. The man they had seen was my brother with his wife on their way to Lamaze class! Nursing is in the Miracle Moments!

Kathy Medenwald, RN
Special Care Nursing, San Diego

*"There are only two ways to live your life.
One is as though nothing is a miracle. The other
is as though everything is a miracle."*
Albert Einstein

The Gift

You might think I'm insane to admit openly that a cancer diagnosis at age 37 was a gift from God, but it's true. Well, okay, not initially, because as you might suspect, at first I was as terrified and as sick as is possibly imaginable.

The gift was the process of walking through this experience with the love, support, encouragement and wisdom of an army of individuals who saved my life on many levels. One of those individuals not only saved my life but also saved my spirit.

As I mentally prepared myself for each grueling, six-hour chemotherapy session, I would struggle with thoughts of should I or shouldn't I go through with it, as Lord only knows which body part would fall off as a result, as if losing my hair, eyebrows and back teeth were not enough.

Not to mention the thought of toxic waste pumping through my body and the residual effects ranging from feeling like death on a bad day to feeling a little less dead on a good day. Through it all, though, one person kept me coming back for another round—Dr. Matthew Cohen, Chief of Service, Behavioral Health, Kaiser Permanente Woodland Hills.

Dr. Cohen is an exceedingly compassionate man and without my ever asking him, he managed to take time out of his hectic schedule and spend time with both my husband and me. He never missed a round. It was his smile, quick wit, kind gestures and calming presence that motivated me to remain hopeful and believe that this journey was a lesson in life that I needed to endure and would preserve.

To this day, I am not certain that Dr. Cohen realizes the gift of life he gave me through his effortless kindness and compassion. I will forever be grateful and hold him in my heart with high esteem and admiration.

SallyAnn Cross, LCSW
Department Administrator, Addiction Medicine Services, Woodland Hills

"Wherever there is a human being,
there is an opportunity for a kindness."
Seneca

The Epitome of Care

As I lay motionless on the CT table, fear gripped me and tears began to roll down my cheeks. The paging system blared, "ER team to the CT room STAT!" I heard a flurry of activity as the CT scanner room filled with familiar ER staff. They quickly assessed me and then said that they were going to move me onto the gurney and admit me to the hospital. The ER physician, Dr. Lynn, grasped my hand softly, squeezed it, and whispered in my ear, "We're going to take good care of you. We'll get this all sorted out." Then his hand gently wiped away the still flowing tears.

As an active 28-year-old ER nurse, I hardly expected to be the object of an emergency code. While undergoing a chest CT to investigate a variety of troubling symptoms, I had an allergic reaction to the dye. I rapidly developed hives and near complete muscle paralysis due to the drug reaction and my yet to be diagnosed disease process.

I had experienced a two-year history of intermittent fatigue and muscle weakness which often included difficulty breathing, speaking, chewing and swallowing, walking, and holding my head up. I also had fluctuating fatigue, blurred and double vision, and drooping eyelids. Following the injection of the CT dye, I felt warm and itchy almost immediately, my chest became heavy and I couldn't get in a full breath. I was unable to move my head, arms or legs. I couldn't even open my eyes. My vain attempts to call for help were only whispered, unintelligible, slurred speech that no one could understand.

Lab tests along with the CT scan confirmed a diagnosis of myasthenia gravis, a chronic neuromuscular disease. Major chest surgery to remove my enlarged thymus gland was scheduled. I still remember the soft-spoken, gray-haired thoracic surgeon, sitting at the foot of my bed, patting my hand before leaving and saying, "I know you are going to do great, Jeanne."

Before surgery, profound muscle weakness caused my arm and leg movements to be jerky and uncoordinated. My nurses taught me several ways to communicate that didn't involve too much talking and we had good two-way communication using a letter board to relay my needs. I would have starved if it had not been for the kind assistance of the dietary and nursing staff helping me to feed myself.

After each meal, food had fallen onto my sizable bib, my bed and even onto the floor. As the housekeeping staff cleaned up my stray food, they showed their kindness by asking me about my family. They took the time to encourage me and several joked that they would see me again after my next meal. The humor and caring of the whole health care team was the perfect medicine to treat my fear and anxiety.

After chest surgery, another host of health professionals supported my gradual recovery. The pain was intense, but I still had to move, take deep breaths and try to feed myself. The nurses made sure I was medicated so I could participate fully with all therapies and be as comfortable as possible, even with all the tubes!

I could barely see my caregivers through my droopy eyelids and blurred vision, but their gentle touches and the warmth in each familiar voice was always reassuring. Respiratory therapists popped in often, greeted me warmly, and rallied my best efforts during treatments with enthusiastic cries of, "Okay, now draw in a big breath, more, more, more, a little bit more. Great job!" They knew this therapy was critical to preventing a life-threatening pneumonia.

My confidence was built as skilled physical therapists competently retrained my wobbly muscles to move and walk in a more coordinated way. I learned how to eat safely without choking, while conserving my limited strength and energy from friendly occupational therapists.

I fondly remember the genuine patience and compassion shown by each member of the health care team as they supported my struggle to relearn old skills or refine new skills throughout my recovery. Their efforts came together beautifully like pieces of a uniquely designed quilt, each skill, encouraging word, and gentle touch became an essential part of my eventual physical and emotional recovery.

Jeanne Rhynsburger, RN, MBA
Ambulatory Care Practice Leader II, Lancaster

"The central concerns of nursing—care, comfort, guidance, and helping individuals cope with health problems—have not changed."
Eleanor Lambertsen

Divine Intervention

It was an ordinary, busy day at the Mission Viejo Nurse Clinic. I was working hard to keep my patients healthy and happy. I glanced outside and spotted my dear patient Mr. Russell. He came in daily for wound care, but on this visit, I observed him as very diaphoretic.

I brought him back to an exam room to assess him. A low blood pressure was unusual for him. He was pale and complained of dizziness. I decided to take him to urgent care for a physician evaluation. His vital signs showed that he required admission to the hospital.

He refused to go. I silently prayed that he would change his mind. I feared that he might cause an accident, possibly injuring himself or others. While monitoring him in the urgent care clinic area, his blood pressure became critically low and they called 911. The paramedics took him to the hospital where he remained for five days. He had overdosed on beta-blockers.

After his stay in the hospital, he returned to thank me for intervening on his behalf when he was feeling so ill. Mr. Russell asked what I had done or said to him to change his mind about the hospital admission. I told him that it was a much higher power that had made that decision.

Subsequently, after a continued month of dressing changes on his wound, it healed with no other complications. I will always remember this as a tragedy we avoided here at Mission Viejo Medical Office.

Beny Tadina-Himes, RN
Mission Viejo Medical Office, Orange County

"Nurses are angels in comfortable shoes."
Author Unknown

Don't Forget to Smile

When I look back on my career choice, I can't actually visualize the moment I decided to become a nurse. But, when I ask myself now why I chose it, the answer is easy. Being a nurse isn't something I do, it is something I am.

I have met so many wonderful people since I entered this profession. Each and every one of them made an impression on me, and some of them had a huge impact. I have worked in many different areas of nursing, and each one presented different challenges and generated different rewards. While saving lives may seem the most exciting, I actually find my current role as a senior nurse in family practice the most rewarding.

Family practice is the area of medicine that encompasses the entire spectrum of life. Starting from the two-day newborn visit, I have watched families grow. At the other end of the spectrum are the elderly patients that I see daily. Many of my families are multigenerational. I see people every day whose lives I have touched and who have touched mine.

The person that I will remember most was a patient who developed ovarian cancer at the age of 49. She worked as a receptionist and greeted all the people that came into the clinic with a smile. She had such a joy for life and always took challenges in stride.

When she first became ill, she worked part-time and was a very active volunteer in the community. During the course of her three-year battle, she never stopped helping other people. She took time off when she started her chemotherapy, but went right back to work as soon as she could.

She always looked to the future. She said, "I am going to get better and get back to work," and she did. She was able to come back several times, and every time she returned, it was with that beautiful smile. She engaged even the grumpiest person in conversation.

She was so grateful for every day that she had. It never bothered her that she was bald, skinny or tired all the time. She lived every second. She faced her disease and her life with strength of character, optimism and joy. She passed that joy on to everyone around her.

I was fortunate to visit her in the hospital two days before she died. She was concerned about her family and about how they would get along without her. She had come to terms with her imminent death and had made peace with the fact that she wasn't going back to work this time. The last thing she said to me was, "Don't forget to keep smiling."

Her funeral was standing room only. Family, friends, coworkers, community members and even patients came to pay respects to this woman. Whenever I feel myself forgetting to smile, I stop and think about her. I think about how easily she could have given up, but she didn't. How easily she could have wallowed in self-pity, but she didn't. I think about how her visits didn't leave me feeling sad that she was dying, but glad that I had known her. That is the reason I am a nurse.

M. Kenne Kennedy, RN
Family Practice, Woodland Hills

"Death ends a life, not a relationship."
Robert Benchley

Returning

I have been a hospice nurse for 14 years. I have cared for many people and have seen and done a great deal in that time. I have many tales I could tell, but some just seem to stay with me more than others do.

The wife had preceded her husband in death by almost a year and a half. Before she died, she promised him that she was going to come back as a hummingbird so she could watch over him.

Miraculously, one and a half months before her husband's death, a hummingbird built a nest in a ficus tree outside his window. The nest had broken bits of eggshells. They were turquoise, his wife's favorite color.

The hummingbird had two babies that brought much delight and comfort to the husband and his three daughters. His wife had kept her promise. She was in close proximity and watching over them.

This story was told at the husband's memorial.

Susan F. Romo, RN
Hospice/Home Health, Los Angeles

"There are two ways of spreading light: to be the candle or the mirror that reflects it."
Edith Wharton

Memories

At 13, she hadn't decided what to do with her life. There were so many choices and endless possibilities. This was the 60s; a woman could be more than a housewife.

In the Girl Scouts, with her troop, she was exploring many opportunities. That year along with several other scouts, and joined by a few moms, hers included, she volunteered at the local convalescent hospital wheeling elderly residents to church services held in the recreation room.

The place smelled awful, full of undefined odors. Often, as she transported people she'd catch whiffs of old urine and sour antibiotics. But their delighted, hopeful faces kept her coming back every Sunday in her scout uniform instead of attending her own church with her family and friends.

It was a large institution. The best part was getting to talk to these survivors of life on the long walk to and from the recreation room. They were living history books. The men told tales of wars, hopping trains, driving trucks, building bridges, and sometimes of spouses lost or sons and daughters who were coming to visit soon.

The women talked of their families, lost husbands, their children, especially their children. They often shared stories about their favorite nurses and doctors because they knew the scouts were considering careers in health care.

"I remember the first one," she said. "I was so young. It was different back then. They never told the young girls anything, thinking not to worry us. We were supposed to trust the doctors.

"My husband and I were so scared," she said as she was pushed along in her wheelchair. "We didn't know what to expect. We had

stayed in California after the war and my mother was back east.

"They made Johnnie stay in the waiting room and they put me in a room with another lady who was moaning," she said. "But my nurse, Rosie, was so kind. Right away, she smiled at me and made me feel safe. 'I'll be with you the whole time. Don't worry.'

"Rosie explained everything, what would happen, how I would feel, how she would always be with me," she said. "Rosie told me we'd do it together.

"I was supposed to have a 'saddle block' for the delivery," she went on. "The doctor came at the last minute and was upset because I couldn't stop laboring so he could do it.

"I cried because I was trying the best I could," she said. "Rosie was with me, though. She whispered into my ear that everything was fine and I was doing a great job. Then she stood right up to my doctor and told him what was what!

"Suddenly, the baby came!" she said. "The doctor was still upset because I tore and he had to sew me up. But Rosie said I had done everything right and he was just being grouchy.

"When he left, Rosie wrapped my baby in a cotton blanket and let me hold him. We could have gotten in trouble because that was against the rules back then. But Rosie stood guard at the door so I could. He was so beautiful, my first son. I have never forgotten Rosie," she said.

I collected many stories that year. I was impressed by how many elderly women were confused and forgetful about the present, but could remember minute details about the far past, frequently about their childbirth experiences and the nurses who cared for them.

Their reverence for these nurses inspired me to choose a nursing career for myself, specializing in maternal-child health.

Luci Eversole, RNC, MSN

Clinical Director, Maternal-Child Health/Nursing Administration, Fontana

"What is history? An echo of the past in the future; a reflex from the future on the past."

Victor Hugo

A Long Shot

Andrew was in his mid 30s and had leukemia when we met. He qualified for home health care because he was too weak to go into the clinic for his routine chemotherapy or get his blood drawn prior to treatment. I became his home health nurse.

I saw Andrew at least once a week to care for his central line, draw his labs, give his chemotherapy, and/or transfuse blood products. Occasionally, he would be hospitalized for neutropenic fever, but he usually bounced right back.

After several weeks of caring for him, it became more and more predictable when he would need hospitalization and when he would need a transfusion. In fact, my projected schedule would include a day when he was my only patient because of the time it took to give him a blood transfusion.

After several hospitalizations, Andrew asked me if I could help him "get conditioned" so he could take his wife on a cruise for their 10th wedding anniversary. The cruise was going to last one week.

We both knew that if he took his chemotherapy the week prior to leaving that he would not likely make the trip. According to our usual schedule, he'd be due for his blood transfusion the week of the cruise. We had to think out of the box.

It was a long shot but I convinced Andrew's oncologist to give his blood transfusion one week early and hold his chemotherapy for the week. Andrew went on the cruise and had a "blast" according to his wife.

He came back weaker than ever and once again needed hospitalization. This time, however, he did not come home. I think, though, he must have died happy.

Gemma Frulla, RN, MSN
Home Health, San Diego

*"Caring is a reflex. Someone slips, your arm
goes out. A car is in the ditch, you join the
others and push...You live, you help."*

Ram Dass

In a Blink

Iremember the year. It was 1988. I was a nursing student from Cypress College doing my maternal-child health rotation in L&D. I was so excited. Kaiser Permanente employed nurse-midwives and I wanted to be one. I met Ilene Gelbaum, CNM, that day after watching her deliver a baby. I remember as though it was yesterday. I ran down the hall after her, calling out, "I want to be just like you!"

Fast forward to 1989 when Kaiser Permanente Anaheim offered me a position on the surgical orthopedic floor. I spent the next two and a half years growing as a new nurse. I worked nights, soaking up all the experiences and lessons of the seasoned nurses. In the blink of an eye, I was a primary nurse.

Another blink and I transferred to postpartum. I loved teaching new moms, but I wanted more. Eight months later, I proposed the idea of transferring to L&D if I took L&D and fetal monitoring classes at my own expense. To my satisfaction, the answer was yes!

Blink! Night shift, 1992 and I walked through the L&D doors with purpose. I was both excited and scared. What was I thinking? My lifelong dream was to be a midwife, but I had never even been pregnant! I remember taking a deep breath and hanging onto everything the L&D nurses taught me. Without them, their patience and wisdom, I would not have succeeded. I met some wonderful women in L&D. One became my best friend. Another became my mentor and guide.

The midwives were awesome. They were all so very different: different backgrounds, different training, but solidly united in their care of women. I was inspired and worked hard as a nurse in L&D. Ilene and I delivered many babies together. I continued to tell her I wanted to be just like her.

Blink! Summer 2000 and I was finishing my BSN at California State University,

Los Angeles (CSULA). Every time that I mentioned that I wanted to become a midwife, I got back nothing but encouragement. BJ Snell, CNM, a per-diem midwife at Kaiser Permanente Anaheim, was also the director of the midwifery program at the University of Southern California (USC). Pennie Darnell, CNM, told me BJ had just announced the USC program was looking for applicants. It was seemingly impossible, due to financial concerns, but it deserved a try.

Blink! I applied to the USC midwifery program. They accepted me! Not even done with my CSULA finals and I was on my way. I started USC with awe and amazement. There I was taking lecture notes in a master's level class one day, and then taking my undergraduate finals the next day. When something is meant to be, mountains move. It felt like God called me. Okay, maybe not called, YELLED!

Blink! December 2001 and I successfully graduated from USC with my certificate in midwifery and a master's degree. Blink again. Kaiser Permanente Anaheim, my first choice, hired me as a midwife. Now, six years and close to 700 deliveries later, when Ilene introduces me to her patients, she still jokingly tells them that she taught me everything I know.

The women I have had the privilege to care for have left indelible imprints on my heart. I can't remember all of them, but many stand out. It is a blessing to care for and deliver women with their second, third, and even fourth pregnancies. It is an honor, and a good reason to work as hard as I do, when my patients request to see only me. Mix that together with the fact that I am part of a fantastic group of women who are my colleagues. It adds up to success. My dream to be a certified nurse-midwife came true, in a blink.

Laura Garcia-Lance, CNM, MSN

OB/GYN, Orange County

"Go confidently in the direction of your dreams.
Live the life you've imagined."

Henry David Thoreau

Loving One Another

In over 36 years of professional nursing, I have lived many stories with patients and their families. This story is about a member of my Kaiser Permanente family. I believe it speaks to the compassionate presence of love in the midst of pain and suffering.

Albert was in his thirties. He was a coworker and the lead x-ray technician on the night shift. His manner was quiet with a huge smile. He approached each patient by introducing himself and putting the patient at ease before doing the x-ray. Before he shot the film, he announced in a clear voice, "X-ray, last call" so the staff was not exposed to the radiation.

Albert began to experience pain in his side and asked one of the physicians to do an MRI to clarify the cause of the discomfort. The MRI detected pancreatic cancer. Albert took a leave of absence to attend to his health. The news of his diagnosis devastated us.

"It isn't fair," one of us said. "He is such a nice guy."

"Albert doesn't deserve this," said another. "I can't believe this is happening."

Comments such as these were heard throughout the unit as we attempted to digest what was happening to our colleague. We shared our feelings and consoled each other as best we could. Then we took action and collected more than $700. We wrote personal notes and cards to Albert including our prayers and good wishes. We underscored how much he was missed at work too.

In response, Albert sent the following thank-you card to us:

> To all the cardiac surgery unit nurses and staff:
> First, let me apologize for not having the strength to write each

and everyone of you individually as I would like to, but the chemo-therapy has left me a little weak and I hope you will forgive me for this.

I was nothing less than overwhelmed as I kept opening the different cards, reading your words and finding money and checks. By the time I opened the last card, I was in tears and so grateful to have friends like you in my life!

When I found out about my condition and that my days were most likely numbered, I began to wonder if my life had made any difference at all. After receiving your cards I felt so loved and missed that I knew I must have done something right. So, thank you for giving me this, "It's A Wonderful Life" moment when I needed it the most. And if this is my "Last Call" please know that you have shed a warm light on what would have otherwise been the darkest time in my life.

With all my love, Albert

Lynne Romanowski, RN
Cardiac Surgery Unit, Los Angeles

"When we share—that is poetry in the prose of life."
Sigmund Freud

Just Doing My Job

As a nurse, one must sometimes ask the questions, am I really helping people to the best of my ability? Do people really care what we, as nurses do? Not too long ago, I received answers to my questions and I was very delighted at the response brought to me by a patient and his family.

In critical care, we take care of many types of patients and it is extremely satisfying to see many of them get better. Sometimes, however, people are so ill or injured that they die. Death does not discriminate; it can be anyone, young or old, male or female. One particular eye-opening experience left me thankful that I am a critical care nurse and happy in my job.

This patient was very sick and received emergent intubation. He was dying. We notified his family who immediately started calling other members of the family. By the time everyone had arrived, the patient was gravely ill, but more stable.

We called a family meeting. It moved from the bedside to a conference room because of the large number of relatives present. By my count, more than 15 family members had gathered with two more in attendance by speakerphone.

I, along with the doctor, discussed the patient's serious prognosis with the family. We informed them of all the options available. Decisions about the patient's quality of life had to be made. They were all asking many questions and were trying hard to decide what to do. Ultimately, they requested more time to notify other family members and because other relatives were on the way to the hospital.

The doctor left and I remained in the conference room with the family. I let them know that whatever decision they made, I would make sure that their father/grandfather was not in any pain and would be comfortable. He was my patient and my priority, I told them. They hugged me and thanked me.

They had only one request, that when the rest of the family arrived, they wanted to gather at the bedside as a group. I told them that once their father/grandfather was off the ventilator that would be possible. They could be together for his last moments.

After several hours, the family came to a decision. They knew he would not want to live on a machine. They asked us to remove the ventilator. Then the family could be together peacefully.

When the family entered the critical care unit, I was astonished. People kept coming in. They did not stop. They were very courteous and quiet, even the several young children. I counted nearly 40 people in the patient's room.

The room was very small but moving the equipment out of the way allowed the entire family to be at the bedside. It brought tears to my eyes to see such love and support. I stepped away and let them pray in peace.

When his heart finally stopped, a few relatives came up to me and thanked me for giving them the opportunity to be together at this sad time. They were so close and they did not want their father/grandfather to die alone. They wanted him to die surrounded by his family. They were so thankful that I granted them this wish. I get emotional when I think of them or whenever I pass by the room where he died.

The next day I received a call from the unit that a special delivery had arrived for me. The family sent me a fabulous bouquet of flowers. I could not believe it. I started to cry. This family had just experienced a great loss yet they were thanking me and I was just doing my job.

Enclosed with the flowers were two beautiful notes, one from the children and one from the grandchildren. They thanked me for helping them through this rough time in their lives and for going beyond their expectations. Yet, I was just doing my job.

I love my work and I will never have to doubt that again. People really do care, and I am glad to be doing what I do. I am a nurse. My primary focus is caring for the sick and the injured. Some say it is a thankless job, but I think it is a thankful job.

Stephanie C. Zarate, RN
Critical Care, Baldwin Park

"If you have not often felt the joy of doing a kind act, you have neglected much, and most of all yourself."
A. Neilen

Machines

We used to take pulses
Instinctively feeling
Just the right spot
On the inner wrist

Now we use machines.

We used to feel
Warmth
Or a dry coolness
And an energy that
Kept time
Precisely
Or lost its way
Changing rhythms
Indecisively

Now we use machines.

We sometimes crept into the
    sleeping room
Watched quietly for respirations
And stealthily felt the heart's
Rhythm without waking anyone
Touching a person so simply
Gave us so much

It gave us
A way to know their strength
Their weakness
Their ability to trust
And their acceptance of our touch

Machines.

Marilyn Mitchell, RN, BSN
Education Consultant, Education and Consulting Services, San Diego

Misery is Optional

I worked in the Department of Preventive Medicine at Kaiser Permanente San Diego for many years. One of the most memorable patients I saw was a young woman in her early 30s, by the name of Angel.

Her poise, grace and sweet demeanor struck me. I had reviewed her chart prior to seeing her, and since the visit was for a comprehensive health evaluation, there was a section on psychosocial history. It was clear just from the chart review that she had experienced a very troubled, abusive childhood.

When I was interviewing her, I was shocked to learn that she had suffered just about every possible kind of abuse. Yet one would never suspect such a background because she presented so serene and composed.

She was a dramatic contrast from the many patients I had seen who carried so much tragic baggage from disturbed pasts, addictive behaviors, serious health consequences and multiple somatic complaints.

I asked her what had been the key that enabled her to move past the pain of all she had endured. How had she become the picture of health, not just in the physical sense, but also in the psychosocial sense?

She answered simply, "My faith in God but also an adage that I live by, 'Pain is inevitable but misery is optional.' I chose not to be miserable."

I had never heard those words before and remarked that I loved that saying. I wanted to write it down and frame it for my exam room so I could share it with other patients. She replied that she was taking a calligraphy course and would be happy to do it for me.

True to her word, I soon received it in the mail, set in a lovely frame, with her first name in the lower left corner. It has been in the rooms where I see my patients ever since. Many people have commented on it through the years. Hopefully, it has inspired them to choose hope and not misery.

Carolyn Ball, PA-C
Population-Based Medicine, San Diego

"We are made wise not by the recollection of our past, but by the responsibility for our future."
George Bernard Shaw

Sunshine

During my first year as a newly graduated nurse, I found myself back in the classroom for a three-month orientation, hitting the books again and looking at patients from a distance. With that instruction under my belt, I started my clinical rotations which included a month in each unit.

One of my first rotations was in the ER. A young tennis pro, close to my age, presented in excellent health, except for an inexplicable case of jaundice. I worked with him for the majority of the day. As nice as I tried to be, we did not bond.

"Not one of his better days," I told myself in an attempt to explain away his negative behavior. My next month-long rotation took me to the Cardiac Cath Lab, where I soon forgot my days in the ER, and moved on to other challenges. "Maybe this specialty is the right fit for me," I thought.

About seven weeks after my encounter with my young, sick patient in the ER, I saw him again, only this time, he was sedated, intubated and had progressed to a unique shade of yellow. His change in health was so dramatic—from athletic and successful to very sick and frail.

His father was by his side almost every day. He was my assignment for the entire month of my ICU rotation because of the opportunities his care presented with dialysis, invasive cardiac monitoring and other treatments. I was slated as a one-to-one, so I could provide full 12-hour bedside care, which he needed.

The following month found me in the CCU. Again, I was sure I had found my calling. I loved the pathway of the fresh heart patient. Then, I was off to the Neuro-ICU where lo and behold, I met my friend again. This time, he was unrecognizable, except for the name on the door. After a few months in the hospital, patients can transform.

I cared for him for another month through total sedation, more tests and invasive, life-sustaining therapies. Fortunately, my patient showed some signs of improvement, and was transferred back to the Medical-Surgical ICU with hopes of making it to Intermediate Care once he was weaned from the ventilator.

I met up with him again in Intermediate Care about six weeks later. I was pleasantly surprised when I got to the unit on my first day and saw his name on the door. I asked my mentor if I could take him as a patient. She giggled and looked at me with a huge grin. "Sure," she said. "Why don't you call me when you need me?"

I didn't know that he had gained a reputation of being a difficult patient. I walked into his room feeling very excited to see him with his eyes open. I learned very quickly that he was the same grumpy person I had cared for that first day in the ER.

When his father arrived, he recognized me and told his son about my role in his care starting from day one and spanning what was now approaching seven months. From that point on, he was more compliant and accepting but we had not achieved "welcoming."

I volunteered to take him for the next week and was soon the hero of the unit. We began to form a friendship. We started to talk about some of the care he received when he was not aware of his surroundings. The loss of time and absence of place had frustrated him tremendously.

One day, I had the task of taking him to CT. I needed the help of my mentor to place him on a monitor and wheel him down on a gurney for the scan. When we got off the elevator on the first floor, I stopped the gurney and asked my patient, "When was the last time you had the sun on your face?"

He had no time to respond before my mentor stopped me and said, "No. We can't take him outside."

"Why not," I said. "He's on the monitor, we have no cause to think he's in any danger, and the door is very close to us."

My patient looked at the senior nurse and said, "Please." She relented and out we went.

It was an amazingly clear, sunny, warm fall day. Seven months after the day he had walked through what might have been a one-way door, we stood there with the sun shining on our faces. Tears filled my patient's eyes. My mentor relaxed. I sensed she too had a moment of reflection about her long, industrious career.

I had really hoped that I could make a difference for my patient. From my vantage point, it looked like the care that I had provided during his long hospitalization had helped facilitate his recovery. In that instant, I realized that the Medical-Surgical ICU was where I wanted to be.

I was off on the day of his discharge. I heard they had a celebration; it was not because an ornery patient was leaving, but because of his successful recovery. Those few moments of sunshine changed him. He had a reason to get better. He missed being outdoors and wanted more of it. He was nicer to everyone from that day forward and progressed quite rapidly.

Imagine my holiday schedule that first year of nursing. There I was working the Christmas Eve night shift in my new home away from home, the Medical-Surgical ICU, when a vaguely familiar young man came in through the unit door.

I attempted to place him. Then I noticed his eyes and remembered the day when I saw them open for the first time in Intermediate Care. It was him. He walked up to me, handed me a dozen roses and hugged me.

"Thank you for giving me the motivation I needed to get well and get out of the hospital," he said. He told me that it was the sunshine that he had always taken for granted that he missed the most. "Seeing it again gave me the drive to recover," he said.

That was the most amazing Christmas of my life, and the best gift a nurse could ever receive. For me, that experience became my guiding light in nursing practice. I love what I do, and I will always remember how it is the little things that we do that make such a difference.

Tracy Abrams, RN, MSN

Assistant Department Administrator, Quality Assurance, San Diego

"Nursing encompasses an art, a humanistic orientation, a feeling for the value of the individual, and an intuitive sense of ethics, and of the appropriateness of action taken."

Myrtle Aydelotte

Humbled

Evening shift as a nurse anesthetist is totally unpredictable, you never know what you are going to be doing. One evening in OR1, I had the satisfaction of working with a patient from ICU emergently needing anesthesia for a bowel obstruction.

The pre-op workup was on the spot. The patient was short of breath but awake. I interviewed him, looking him in his eyes. I had only a few minutes to build that trust factor that is so important before receiving anesthesia.

When I was done, I asked him if he had any questions. He was very sick, with a low blood pressure and needing surgery immediately.

Point blank, without missing a beat, he said, "Am I going to die?" His response took me off guard.

Silence ensued for a long five seconds. My response was caring and truthful. "You are very sick," I said. "But I will do the best I am able to take good care of you."

He had HIV and a history of substance use. "Thanks for treating me like a real person," he said. I was awestruck.

The anesthesia was challenging, but he made it back to the ICU intubated. As I returned to my department, I passed the OR waiting area. The patient's sister was peering out the door looking at me. I stepped inside, obviously guided from above, and introduced myself.

"Is he okay?" she asked.

One more time that night, my response was caring and sincere as I told her honestly that her brother was very sick and might not make it. She hugged me.

"I just wanted to know the truth," she said. "Nobody is saying how sick he is; that he may not survive."

I was humbled. It would have been so easy to let my judgment of others get in the way of my work.

With my patients, I never really know the rest of their stories so I try to do my best without making my own assumptions. I always aim to treat everyone as if he or she were a member of my family.

At that moment, I knew that I had help in being the best I could be for the patient and for his sister. For that gift I am grateful.

Cynthia Plehn, CRNA
Anesthesia, Los Angeles

"Remember that everyone you meet is afraid of something, loves something and has lost something."
H. Jackson Brown, Jr.

A Grandmother's Story

Being a nurse is great and rewarding. But, being a Catholic nurse and totally pro-life can be challenging, especially when I have to write abortion referrals. However, regardless of my personal beliefs, I act professionally. I have learned to keep my thoughts to myself unless a patient asks for my advice.

A woman came in for a routine blood pressure check. Her 19-year-old daughter had just found out she was pregnant. The young girl was in her second year of college. She had graduated from high school with honors and had a full scholarship to attend California State University, Northridge.

She was the oldest of four children and expected to be a good example for her younger siblings. When she found out she was pregnant, she called her mother to discuss her decision to have an abortion. Her mother thought that abortion was not the solution, but decided to support her daughter's choice.

On that afternoon, as we talked, she opened her heart. She told me about her daughter and asked me what I thought. I was cautious. I asked her permission to share my own personal experience and then added my coworker's story whose daughter also got pregnant in college but decided to keep the baby. The young mother went on to finish school and marry the father.

The woman shared her religious beliefs with me and asked me to pray for her daughter. I promised I would.

A few months later, someone knocked on the door to my department. When I opened it, the woman rushed in. Filled with joy, she hugged me and then started crying.

"I am going to be a grandmother," she said. "I am here to thank you. You are the reason my daughter decided to keep her baby. She is due to deliver in a few more weeks."

The woman shared with me that her daughter was engaged to the baby's father and they were planning their wedding after their baby's birth. They both remained in college. In my mind, I knew God had touched her daughter's heart and that I had made a difference in her life.

Angela Morones, RN
Nurse Visit Clinic, Palmdale

*"Kind words can be short and easy to speak,
but their echoes are truly endless."*
Mother Teresa

Dad

From a patient letter

My story is really one about my dad, Murray Kray who died on May 16, 2008 from pneumonia. (He also had dementia.) My dad was a strong advocate of Kaiser Permanente. He joined in the early 50s when he and my mother had small children. Kaiser Permanente took great care of us then and continues to do so now. But, the most important part of my dad's story is the way he was cared for as he aged.

At every juncture of my dad's health history, the people of Kaiser Permanente stepped up and treated his various conditions completely. From bypass surgery to prostate problems, cataracts and cancer, they handled each issue with great care and compassion.

As his daughter and health care giver, most significant was the way that the Woodland Hills Geriatric Department took care of my dad as he started showing signs of dementia. The approach of the team was stellar and included Dr. Mason, Dr. Chandra, Netta (his pharmacologist) and Deborah Wilkes (his social worker). This group went so far beyond his ordinary day in and day out care that I had to write this letter. Even the reception people in this department were great.

My dad and our family were treated with dignity and caring. We always received return phone calls as well as appointments and follow-ups whenever needed. The fact that this highly specialized care exists as it does at Kaiser Permanente Woodland Hills is extraordinary. But, even more so, the people who deliver the care are wonderfully compassionate and competent.

This team helped to complete the circle of my dad's life. In the end, when we decided on hospice for him, Deborah Wilkes and Dr. Chandra went into action and made sure that he had whatever he needed for his care. Dr. Chandra reached out to us as a family and really impressed us with the way he was there for my dad.

I just wanted to express my thanks to Kaiser Permanente for providing this end-of-life experience and for keeping my dad healthy as long as they could.

Thank you so much.

Janet Scharf
Account Executive, Kaiser Brand Store, Woodland Hills

"There are no traffic jams
when you go the extra mile."
Attributed to both Zig Ziglar and Dr. Kenneth McFarland

Surrounded and Connected

My story took place in February 2000 when I received a diagnosis of cancer of the esophagus. At that time, I had been a therapist in the Physical Therapy Department at Kaiser Permanente Woodland Hills for 10 years. My patients had a variety of diagnoses but most of them were stroke survivors.

One of my patients was a 77-year-old woman with very strong family support and spiritual convictions. They were totally committed to her survival and never missed an appointment with me. Therapy was difficult for her because it was exhausting and intense. Yet she made her best effort because her family encouraged her. I saw her every week in my Stroke Survivor's support group after her discharge from physical therapy.

In January 2000, I had a few episodes of food sticking behind my sternum. My regular physician was not available so I asked our worker's compensation physician to see me. I described a general malaise feeling and difficulty getting food down past my sternum. I had not lost any weight so there did not seem to be a concern but she ordered an x-ray and a swallow study. She called me after she received the results and said she needed to see me right away.

I went to her office and she told me I had a two-centimeter tumor behind my sternum at the junction between the esophagus and the stomach. I was in shock. She scheduled me for an immediate endoscopy and then said, "Bonnie, these tumors are malignant."

I had no clue. Cancer does not run in my family. My parents were healthy and in their 70s. There was not even a single case of breast cancer among my relatives.

The next day, the endoscopy confirmed adenocarcinoma of the esophagus. I went through the usual scenarios in my head. I wanted to be around to raise my children, retire with my husband and have a full life. I never thought cancer would be my fate.

I met with my supervisor. I told her about my diagnosis and that I would be out for several months to undergo treatment. I did not know how it would end. She supported me every step of the way. She had a heart of gold along with her trademark compassion. Ultimately, she became my role model as I moved on to manage others.

I told my patients that I would be out for awhile but other therapists would fill in for me. The rest of the department heard about my diagnosis, formed prayer circles and sent weekly cards to keep my spirits up. Then my treatment began.

I had a PICC line inserted so I could receive my chemotherapy, cysplatin (a five-hour IV drip) and 5FU (which I received 24 hours a day for seven days) over the course of eight months at the Woodland Hills Medical Center. I had five weeks of radiation therapy and my surgery at the Los Angeles Medical Center.

On a visit to the Woodland Hills Medical Center, a receptionist said that one of my former patients wanted to contact me and asked if that would be okay. I said yes. Soon after, the patient's daughter called. I had taken such good care of her mother that the family would like to take care of me while I was going through cancer treatments.

It turns out the lovely 77-year-old woman who had survived a stroke had two daughters working at the Los Angeles Medical Center. One of them was a pre-op nurse and the other was an anesthesiology nurse. I took this as a sign that everything would be all right. These two nurses would be my guardian angels that would see me through my surgery.

Radiation was easy. Chemotherapy was uncomfortable and left mouth sores, nausea and fatigue but the surgery proved to be the hardest part of the treatment. It was difficult to walk, the chest tubes at the surgery site caused great pain and the inability to have food for seven days was tough.

Before I could eat again I had to go through a swallow study that inverted me to make sure there were no leaks from the surgery. It was tough to hold down the liquid without a valve and everything was backing up into my throat, but I did it. I just took one moment at a time and dealt with it. I could not look at the big picture because it was overwhelming. I did not know where the road would lead.

I felt that ultimately, it was the community of people—my family and friends, coworkers and patients, social workers, nurses and physicians—who surrounded me, encouraged me and kept me connected to life that made a difference in my survival. The quality of care at Kaiser Permanente was world class. I have met other cancer survivors who have reported the same experience.

It has been eight years. In that time I have obtained my Master of Public Health, seen all three of my children graduate from high school and college, and two are enjoying wonderful careers. I have traveled to Europe four times, Israel once and celebrated numerous family functions and holidays. Life is good!

Bonnie J. Weissman, MPH
Department Administrator, Health Education, Physician Education,
Partners in Health, Woodland Hills

"We need four hugs a day for survival.
We need eight hugs a day for maintenance.
We need twelve hugs a day for growth."
Virginia Satir

More Than Required

I was a young new graduate when I started my career with Kaiser Permanente as a per diem radiologic technologist. Soon after, I took the next step in life, marriage. With plans of starting a family, I needed to find a non-per diem job so I accepted a part-time position that offered me training in CT. I was eager to learn, and my wife and I gained the security and benefits that the part-time position offered. I added a plethora of knowledge learned in radiology as well as in the other departments.

The hours I worked were late, long and often varied. After about three years with Kaiser Permanente, my wife and I were expecting our first child. Again, I felt that my job needed to change. Still eager to learn, I wanted to find a position that offered growth as well as hours that were better suited for my new role of husband and father. Soon after, I learned about a great opportunity Kaiser Permanente was offering.

The Director of Southern California Diagnostic Imaging assembled a program that would teach radiologic technologists the specialty of MRI in order to fill the void of much needed positions. The three-month program involved formal studying Monday through Friday, from 8 a.m. to 4 p.m. and I would continue to receive my pay while I was learning. Obtaining an MRI license guaranteed an MRI job.

Unlike CT, MRI is usually staffed during the day. Knowing my situation and the opportunity at hand, my lead technologist urged me to apply for the program. Weeks later, the director of my department gave me the good news that I was accepted.

I started the course when my wife was approximately seven-months pregnant. The director of the program, the instructor, and the other five students (Kaiser Permanente employees) were excited for me, the expectant father. They often teased me. "You will be too busy changing diapers to study," someone would inevitably say.

They were an incredible group. I was ready to do both, but I had no preparation for what really took place.

I received a call from my wife because she was not feeling well. I left class early to meet her at the hospital. She gave birth to my beautiful daughter, who unfortunately was rushed to the NICU. She was suffering from respiratory problems as well as other health issues. She remained in the NICU for two months. It was probably the most difficult eight weeks I had ever experienced.

The physicians could not figure out what was troubling her. Every day was demanding. Many times I wanted to drop out of the program so I could be next to my daughter and wife. While in class, I often felt guilty. The NICU physicians and staff were amazing. Every day at 5 a.m., before leaving to study, I would sit and watch my daughter fight to live.

Not one day passed without someone from the staff placing their hand on my shoulder. Even without words, they spoke to me. Without their comfort, I could not have continued. Every day in class, the group would ask about my daughter and I could sense their concern. The directors of the program and of my department offered their support and help numerous times. If not for their compassion and leniency, I most likely would have dropped out.

My daughter is doing well and I have gained many friends. I completed the MRI program and passed the national licensing exam. I am currently working in MRI with hours that are well-suited for my family's situation.

I cannot be more thankful to those who did more than they were required to do. The compassion that was given to me, I pass on to the patients I care for today. I also feel what many others may never feel, pride in my employer.

Joseph Anthony Azurin
Radiology Technician, Radiology, Bellflower

"Remember there's no such thing as a small act of kindness. Every act creates a ripple with no logical end."
Scott Adams

Lights, Camera, Action

Cindy Baum is a registered nurse who came to Kaiser Permanente West Los Angeles through a traveling agency. She worked in L&D for 13 weeks. When her contract was over, we hired Cindy to fill a vacant position. She was and is an excellent clinician. She was our gain!

Cindy was on duty one weekend when a very anxious husband and wife came into L&D in active labor. During the admission process, the husband was advised that they would be staying.

The husband asked the nurse if he could go back home to get his camera. He told her that he had it ready but forgot to bring it with him when he saw his wife in such pain. Having the camera to record the birth of their baby had been part of their plans for a long time.

Cindy knew that allowing the husband to go back home was not a good idea. His wife was in active labor and he ran the risk of missing the birth altogether. She advised him to stay.

It was the end of Cindy's shift. She left the hospital and purchased a disposable camera from a nearby store. She returned ten minutes before the patient delivered. She handed the camera to the husband who recorded the birth of their beautiful baby boy.

Both the husband and wife could not believe the care, compassion, dedication and, above all, the empathy of this nurse who went beyond the call of duty to provide such a wonderful service.

Because of Cindy's action, I made the decision to purchase disposable cameras and make them available in L&D. We have used them on several occasions because families forgot to bring their own. Based on feedback from many patients and families, having disposable cameras on hand is definitely a plus.

Cindy did not tell anyone about her special deed but the staff observed her dedication and concern. We rewarded Cindy for her special efforts and recognized her for a job so well done.

What a story!

Tessie Furnus Desta, RN, BS, MS
Department Administrator, Perinatal Services, West Los Angeles

*"One of the things I keep learning is that
the secret of being happy is doing things
for other people."*
Dick Gregory

No Kidney Required

It was Thanksgiving Day and I was working the day shift. Normally, I worked in management but decided to give up my day off to work on the floor and allow someone else to be with their family on the holiday.

I walked into a patient's room to hang an IV antibiotic and noticed her IV was pulled out. She was 91 and a little confused. She had been at the skilled nursing facility for three weeks with pneumonia and failure to thrive. Her son was sitting at her bedside watching the football game. I had not seen him before because I normally worked days and he said he usually came in the evenings. But, like me, he had traded his regular shift to help out a friend. We already had something in common.

I made conversation with him as I worked on finding a frail vein to start the IV again. I explained what had happened and what I was doing. Then I asked him where he worked and he told me San Pedro Long Shoring. He glanced at my nametag. "Mattera, you don't look Italian," he said. "You must be Irish or English with that red hair and those green eyes."

"You're right on target. My maiden name was Mitchell," I said then added, "My grandfather worked at the docks."

Then he told me he had worked his job for 37 years. "I probably knew your family," he said.

"Probably not," I said. "My Dad was killed in Vietnam in 1970 and my Grandpa Mitchell died shortly after."

"Mitchell," he said. "I know a Ralph Mitchell."

"I have an Uncle Ralph Mitchell. I haven't seen him in 35 years. Not since my Dad was killed," I said. Nevertheless, my heart began to race. Could this person know my uncle?

Then he said, "Ralph has a brother named Jack."

My heart sank because my other uncle's name was Denny. I doubted it was the same Ralph Mitchell. As I left the room to go on my rounds, I jokingly told the man, "If you find my family, tell them to call me. Tell them I don't need money and there is no kidney required."

Two hours later, the man called his friend Ralph Mitchell. Ralph was awestruck and told him he had two nieces with the same name, Susan Mitchell. "One niece is in Oklahoma. I spoke with her last week," Ralph said. "I haven't seen the other niece in 35 years."

The man told Ralph that I had an uncle named Denny and that my Dad died in 1970 in Vietnam. It was then that Ralph revealed that his younger brother Jack is actually Jack Dennis aka Denny and that his older brother was killed in Vietnam.

My Uncle Ralph called me about three hours later at home. We had a great time catching up and reconnecting. I learned more about my Dad and my family. It became an unforgettable Thanksgiving Day gift.

Often, we as nurses bless others with our acts of compassion, kindness and gentle touch. However, every once in awhile, we are the recipients of caring from those whom we tend.

Susan Mattera, RN, MN
Area Administrator, Home Care, Los Angeles

"Our stories matter...Your stories matter...
For you never know how much of a difference
they make and to whom."
Caroline Joy Adams

A Simple Act of Kindness

I have served as hospital chaplain at Kaiser Permanente South Bay in Harbor City for four years. Until recently, I lived with my family in Hollywood, a 25-mile commute each way through some of the busiest freeways in Los Angeles.

The nature of being a chaplain requires me to be on call 24/7. I can receive a page at any time. I have frequently parked my car in the driveway at home only to receive a page by the family of a seriously ill loved one in need of emergency spiritual care intervention. Often I leave dinner on the table and my family at home in order to return to Harbor City.

I'd had opportunities to work closer to home in the past but I chose instead to continue at South Bay because it is a place I love. I searched for a new house in the South Bay area and, luckily, I was able to find a perfect 3-bedroom home in Harbor City. It was located so close to the medical center campus that I could reach my office within two minutes by car and five minutes on foot.

The house included a swimming pool and spa for my children and a great view with an ocean breeze. My kids could walk to school and I would not have to deal with the strain of traffic or high gas prices. It was perfect but things were about to become even better in ways I could not have even imagined.

I made an offer on the home and the seller accepted it. The agent then arranged for me to meet with the seller for additional negotiations. Before I could introduce myself, one of the women stood up and said, "I know you. You are a chaplain at Kaiser Permanente." I responded affirmatively.

"Two and a half years ago, you prayed for my mother when she died. You came to the room, held our hands and spoke such wonderful words," she said. "We have always remembered you and because of that act of kindness and to thank you, we want to drop the appraised price of this house!" She then added with tears in her eyes that it was her mother's home.

I had no recollection of the family at that moment because I see so many people on any given day. Later, however, I discovered that I did indeed perform the funeral service for her mother. We moved into our house on August 2. My entire family thinks it is unbelievable, awesome and a gift from God. It has been a life-changing experience for all of us.

There is no way to know whom you will meet throughout the day or whose life you will touch in the process. Just because we don't always remember a face or if people you help don't say thank you on the spot, it doesn't mean that our acts of kindness have not touched them.

This experience taught me that people notice what you do and the difference you make in their lives if you do it with sincerity from your heart. As we say in Kenya, mountains do not meet but people do. As we do our best, we never know which life we will touch and we may never know when it will come back to us.

Rev. Joseph Oloimooja, M.Div.
Chaplain, Administration, South Bay

"Kindness is the golden chain by which
society is bound together."
Goethe

A Promise Kept

As nurses, caring is an integral part of us. It encompasses why we chose our profession and how we deliver our touch to each patient we encounter. Our personal and professional lives entwine to enhance the delivery of care every day with every patient we encounter.

My story begins one evening after a heroic effort to save an 18-month-old girl. We lost the battle. I was asked to talk with the mother, since she was physically as well as emotionally unable to relinquish her baby.

As I approached this mom, I knew her grief, anguish, and unfathomable loss because I too had lost my little girls. I felt her pain in the depths of my soul. I felt her agony as the nurse who tried so valiantly to save her baby. Both the nurse and the mom in me grieved with her.

We talked for almost an hour about many things, her baby, her husband on deployment, her loss. I listened and shared a part of me with her. As I looked into her eyes I felt a connection. At that moment I promised her I would personally take care of her little one. She grabbed my hand and again said, "Promise me!" I agreed.

So began the longest emotional journey of my life, taking her little one to the inner depths of our hospital to a morgue that I knew existed but literally had no idea where it was located. I used my nursing skills to gather the information I needed in order to complete my task and then plodded through the corridors to my journey's end.

As I entered the cold and silent room, the employee approached me to hand over the baby. I politely but firmly told the man that I would personally be completing the task.

"I promised her mother," I said to him.

He kindly and gently walked me through each step, helping me to bag and tag appropriately. I did my task with the loving touch of a grieving mom and a caring nurse. As I placed her tiny body on the tray and shut the door, the tears began to flow ever so freely. I grieved for her loss as well as my own.

I had promised a mother to care for her baby until the very end of her journey here on earth. I had kept my promise. Did anyone ever know? Did the mom ever realize the extent of my promise to her? Maybe, maybe not.

As nurses, as Kaiser Permanente nurses, I believe we are measured by the choices we make when no one is looking. Did I make a difference? Yes! Do we make a difference? Yes, we do, every day!

Debra Hill, RN, BSN
Pediatric Clinic, Bellflower

"In compassion lies the world's true strength."
Buddha

She Was Just 13

She was just 13 years old and terrified. In one week she had endured CT scans, MRIs, a biopsy, a tracheostomy, and both a gastrostomy tube and a double lumen Hickman catheter had been placed. These procedures are difficult for anyone but explainable and possibly endurable. But, to this child and her limited understanding due to her developmental delay, all she saw and felt was a strange place with mean people.

Now she had a hole in her belly with a tube sticking out and it was painful. She had another tube from her chest and it hurt too. The hole in her throat made it impossible to talk. She hurt everywhere, she was scared and she wanted to go home, but she couldn't even tell anyone!

Then there was me. I messed with her awful tubes and holes, making her cry but you could hardly hear her screams. I had to give her chemotherapy. I felt so bad for her and I could feel her sense of confusion. Why were they doing all this to her and why weren't her parents making them stop?

I had always spent time with my teen patients. I explained to them the reason they needed the chemotherapy; how it might make them feel, how to get through it and how it was their only chance. I couldn't do this with her but I did my best to explain things in ways she could understand. At first she only cried. All I had to do was enter her room and she would begin to sob.

The first few weeks were tough. I cared for her every day I worked. It was hard for her, the tubes, the pain, the vomiting and then her hair fell out. It was hard for me too, especially knowing how much a positive outlook can make survival so much more likely. I decided I was going to make a difference for her. She needed an ally and I wanted to be that person.

I provided her with the medical care she required, taking meticulous care of her tubes, skin and other physical needs. I pampered her with manicures and pedicures during her baths. Her nails always matched the cute pajamas her mom would bring her. We played with her Barbies and did their hair. I encouraged visits by her friends from school. I tried everything to make her feel like her old self again.

Slowly, we started having some good days. Her doctor would tell me it seemed she was happier and did better when I was there. The first day I saw her smile was a true miracle. My efforts brought her joy but they brought me something more.

She did well throughout the remainder of the very difficult treatment for naso-pharyngeal rhabdomyosarcoma. It is probably one of the toughest to go through involving intensive chemotherapy plus weeks of radiation. But, she was a survivor. Ultimately, she returned to her special education classes with all of her friends, and she was happy.

She is now grown up and doing great. When I see her, I can't help but take pride in the fact that I made a difference for her. She was one of the biggest challenges of my nursing career and by far one of my greatest accomplishments.

Lisa Kanady, RN
Pediatric Oncology, Fontana

*"I am only one; but still I am one. I cannot
do everything, but still I can do something.
I will not refuse to do something I can do."*
Helen Keller

Dave's Legacy

The unthinkable happened four years ago, my brother Dave died from cancer at age 52. As he lay there intubated and unconscious, we, his family, shared our stories and our love for him, laughing and crying. As I watched his blood pressure and heart rate slowly decrease, I wasn't a nurse, I was a sister not fully comprehending what was happening in front of me.

Dave's diagnosis of cancer of the ureter came about three and a half years before he died. It had already metastasized when he had a nephrectomy not long after the discovery of the tumor. He spent his last years "making memories" by traveling and spending time with loved ones. He wasn't bitter or angry and felt that his remaining time was a blessing. In the process of dying, Dave left me his legacy.

He gave me the gift of courage so that I could leave a job I had been in for 26 years to work at Kaiser Permanente. The guts I needed to change jobs seemed so much less than the mettle he needed to face a terminal illness. "Say what you want to say and do what you want to do," he told me.

He gave me the gift of compassion so that I better understand my patients and their families who also face cancer. He taught me that waiting for test results can cause a high level of anxiety and too much information at once can be overwhelming. Displaced anger happens and tears are okay. He showed me that we do not have to know the answers to questions that arise. We only have to listen.

My brother gave me the gift of gratitude. I learned to enjoy and relish the time we have with the people we love. When I hear someone complain about aging, I think that Dave would have been very happy to grow old. He was incredibly grateful for the extra years that he had after his diagnosis.

My brother gave me the gift of acceptance. He was not bitter or angry about the injustice of cancer. I saw that life is not fair but if we spend our time being mad about it, we miss so much. I learned how to harness my anger and use it to create positive action, working for a cause to fight cancer. Otherwise, anger can grow, fester and hurt us.

Losing a loved one is very difficult. But, along with the pain we feel, we can experience happiness from the gifts left to us. For me, they were courage, compassion, gratitude and acceptance. I carry this legacy with me always.

Nancy Elbaum, RN
Outpatient Pulmonary Clinic, Los Angeles

"What you leave behind is not what is engraved in stone monuments, but what is woven into the lives of others."
Pericles

On a Busy Day,
On a Busy Unit

It seemed as if the face of nursing had changed. After 25 years in the profession as a staff nurse and now a manager, I was beginning to feel pessimistic. More and more, I saw nursing focused on the tasks of the day rather than the patient. "Why do we need to teach nurses to give the 'perception' of caring," I began to ask myself. "Why can't we just care?"

I began to feel as though the heart had gone out of nursing practice. I felt like I had lost my belief in nursing as a caring profession until Melinda Guran, RN, and Pearl Olmeda, RN, two nurses on the sixth floor of my hospital, the Medicine-Telemetry Unit, restored my faith.

One extremely busy day, a man was admitted to their unit with abdominal pain. He had a history of pancreatic cancer; it seemed as if it were too late for him. The doctor told him he was not going to make it, he was terminal. In fact, he told him that he probably would not last the day. This poor man had no family in the area. His cousin was coming from out-of-state but would be arriving in the morning, most likely, too late. He was all alone.

Then Mel and Pearl arrived at his bedside. They worked as a team to ensure his comfort, not just for his body but also his spirit. Mel noticed the cross around his neck.

"Are you a Christian?" she asked.

"Yes," he replied. In that instant, Mel recognized his need for more than physical comfort.

"Would you like us to pray with you?" Mel asked.

"Yes," he said.

As Mel and Pearl prayed with this man, time seemed to stop. A look of peace came over him. Mel and Pearl stayed with him, comforting him, holding his hand and praying as his life slowly left him.

This empathy and concern meant a great deal to the patient, to his family and to me. On a busy day, on a busy unit, two nurses, Mel Guran and Pearl Olmeda, took the time to hold a hand, say a prayer and to care.

Both Mel and Pearl are a credit to their chosen profession. They exemplify the heart and soul of nursing and the core value of caring for others. They made me proud to be a nurse again.

Michelle Lane, RN, BSN
Medicine-Telemetry, Orange County

*"I feel the capacity to care is the thing which
gives life its deepest significance."*
Pablo Casals

Communication is Everything

My mother discovered a lump in her breast. She had read that after age 72 it was not necessary to get a mammogram. However, after speaking with a radiology employee, my mother was convinced that she should see her physician.

Her physician referred her for a mammogram, ultrasound and a biopsy all of which happened in one morning and within days of the first doctor visit. Five days later, we received an appointment with a surgeon.

My mother's first language is Spanish. So of course, I asked for an interpreter, who was graciously provided and who was outstanding. The surgeon told us that my mother had breast cancer. We were devastated.

We immediately spoke with the breast cancer coordinator and again had an interpreter. My mother understood everything and was able to ask her questions in her primary language. Having an interpreter present gave my mother a sense of calm. It meant so much to her. Communication is everything!

Seven days from the first visit, she was scheduled for surgery. My mother decided on a mastectomy. We received the same excellent care during pre-op. She even saw a Spanish-speaking physician at the request of the surgeon.

As we checked into SDA, the staff greeted us with smiles and professionalism. As the clerk placed the green wristband I asked the clerk about the color. She explained that green meant my mother needed an interpreter. I was very happy because her language preference was captured in her electronic medical record and anyone who saw her would understand her language needs.

The nursing staff and anesthesiologist were also very good and patient with my mother. After the surgery, my mother stayed in SDA. She slept all night and was very comfortable.

My mother came out of surgery with no pain. She was actually smiling. It was amazing. She was very complimentary towards the SDA nursing staff. For my mother, it was such a positive experience. By the way, she even liked the food.

Six days later, we met with the surgeon and she gave us wonderful news. My mother was cancer free! I am still amazed at how quickly the entire process occurred, from her mammogram to her surgery. All I can say is that our family is very grateful and I am so proud to say that I work for Kaiser Permanente.

Martha A. Brewster
Practice Leader Consultant, SCPMG Executive Offices, Pasadena

"Kind words do not cost much.
Yet they accomplish much."
Blaise Pascal

A Song...Remembered

I cared for a patient admitted to Hospice Services in an advanced state of illness from end stage liver failure. The patient was lethargic, bedridden and completely dependent but I learned a great deal about her through her devoted husband.

One day he told me that she once had a beautiful voice and that the two of them had performed together in the 70s and 80s. Then, much to my surprise and delight, he presented me with a CD recording of them performing.

"You might enjoy listening to this," he said. "It will help you get to know us a little better."

Ironically, I was listening to the music throughout my workday driving between patients, when I received a phone call that she had died. I drove to the house and provided the needed care for her arrangements and support to the husband and other family members.

As I got back in my car, turned on my ignition, the CD music started to play again. She was singing this song:

> Remember me, as like a song
> Sings through your heart and then is gone
> The notes, each played with such delight
> May reach their final chord tonight,
> But like that haunting melody
> Is never gone, will never be.
> Comes back when you are feeling low
> And fills your heart with such a glow
> That cares will fly and in their place

A lighted smile upon your face
All those joys that filled each measure
All those memories we treasure
The notes, each played with such delight
Have found their resting place tonight
Remember me, I am the song
Sings through your heart and then is gone.

"A Song...Remembered"
May 1980

In that most difficult moment, driving away from the house, I experienced her presence in a beautiful and living way through her voice and the heartfelt words of her song. It was as though she had written about her death through this song long before she died.

I have many days filled with difficult and challenging situations and yet, I find that I am often surprised by moments such as this—a fresh and unexpected experience of a person—that carries me through and makes the day extraordinary.

Mary Brennan, RN
Case Manager, Hospice/Palliative Care Programs, Los Angeles

"Our sweetest songs are those that tell of saddest thought."
Percy Bysshe Shelley

A Blessing in My Life

From an in-house publication

When Will Ross carried out his wife's wishes to stop life-sustaining treatments related to her breast cancer, he had the love of his family and friends. He also had support from his care team at Kaiser Permanente Woodland Hills.

"Over the course of Kathy's hospitalization, many of the staff members from the ICU became close to me," said Ross, an administrative judge for the Office of the Secretary of Defense. "They never forgot that Kathy was a person, not just a chart. They treated me, and her, with tremendous compassion and caring."

Since the death of his wife, Kathy Canham Ross, in May 2007, Ross has devoted himself to her memory, helping lead a series of workshops about loss, grief and bereavement for the Woodland Hills ICU staff.

"Bereavement is a difficult topic because no one likes to think about it," said Sharon Kent, ICU Department Administrator, who invited Will to speak to staff members. "We're trying to help our staff understand what it's like to be the person who's going through this painful experience."

The sessions were personally rewarding for Ross. "I can say that the three gatherings were some of the most fulfilling hours of my life since her death," he said. "The questions were probing and searching, and the dialogue was honest.

"What came out of it was that staff members want to help people like me through this time," Ross said. "They want to know what we are feeling and they believe strongly in what they are doing."

Grief is a normal and healthy reaction that occurs when you lose someone or something important. While grief is universal, each person handles emotions and feelings differently.

Support is important during the grieving process. Support comes in many forms, such as from friends and family, by participating in enjoyable activities, or through exercises that express feelings, such as writing letters or keeping a journal.

Ross says he is coping with his wife's death by seeking support from his family and friends and by writing a blog—an online journal—about his emotions. He also receives help from his bereavement support group and John Faas, his medical social worker.

"A support group, at its best—and I go to two great ones—helps us know that we are not alone in what we are feeling in our own separate ways," said Ross.

Fass, a licensed clinical social worker at Kaiser Permanente Woodland Hills, proved an emotional mainstay for Ross as he struggled to deal with the stresses created by his wife's illness and her eventual death.

"Through our sessions, I was able to come to grips with Kathy's death and, ever so slowly, begin to chart the next phase of my life," said Ross. "John has been a blessing to me."

Submitted by:
Sherry Crosby
Public Affairs, Woodland Hills

"We have a choice to use the gift of our life to make the world a better place or not to bother."
Jane Goodall

A Quiet Presence

As a 25-year veteran of Kaiser Permanente San Diego, I have seen and hopefully participated in my share of good deeds, warm thoughts and kind actions. However, because our profession is nurturing and selfless in nature, we don't often allow ourselves to be the recipients of the kindness of others. I learned the true nature of receiving that care some years ago.

I had just given birth to my third son by an unplanned c-section. Unexpectedly, I learned that he had the same autosomal recessive trait that my eldest son had been diagnosed with some 13 years earlier. My new baby was healthy, but not without some known difficulties ahead of him. Joy and elation quickly faded to the "why me, why again?" mantra we are so easily pulled into.

Many colleagues stopped by to offer congratulations and support, but no one compared to Katie Johnson, one of my postpartum nurse friends that I had worked with on the fourth floor.

At 7 a.m., the morning after my son was born, she showed up in my room in scrubs. I thought she was on vacation. It was just three days after Christmas. As the mother of three beautiful daughters, she had earned that time at home with her family. "What was she doing at work, in my room?" I thought.

She gently advised me that she was working, that she was going to "special" me that day. Silly me, I didn't even know what she was talking about. But, I soon found out. She proceeded to disconnect my catheter and IV and helped me out of bed for the first time after my surgery. She helped me bathe, made my bed and sat by my side. She listened to me, wept with me and allowed me to begin to recover physically and psychologically. She helped me begin the emotional healing process.

I will never forget her simple gift of eight hours of her time, vacation time, no less! It seems fitting to share this simple story now. My son just turned 25 years old but it seems like just yesterday.

Katie has since become a perinatal case manager and I am an OB/GYN nurse practitioner. We are both still in the San Diego medical service area. Though our physical paths do not cross as often as they used to, we still speak by telephone when consulting about our patients, and keep up with each other's families.

I will hold the memory of her selfless gift in my heart forever. I try to pass on the gift of unexpected, unasked for caring and compassion in my life and with my patients. Those moments in our lives are truly the "gifts that keep on giving." God bless you, Katie!

Madeline Scull, NP
OB/GYN, San Diego

"It is a beautiful and mysterious power that one human being can have on another through the mere act of caring....A great truth, the act of caring is the first step in the power to heal."
Phillip Moffitt

Pick It Up...Pass It On

I graduated from nursing school in 1981. I was a young and very green new graduate. Sue was the experienced charge nurse of a 40-bed surgical floor, and she was stuck with me on the night shift. I will never forget the night, about six months into my career, when I feel I truly became a nurse.

My 34-year-old patient suddenly developed a GI bleed. Bedpan after bedpan filled with bright red blood and clots. Sue reacted quickly, quietly explaining the procedures to the patient and to me as she started the IV lines.

"Large bore catheters with blood sets," she said. "Two IV lines while you can still get a vein; you can always heparin lock one.

"Use extension tubing so you don't waste time at the catheter hub and maybe lose the line," she calmly told me. "Draw your labs now when you insert the IVs to save a stick 'n' time." My patient actually managed a laugh.

"Ha! I thought that was funny, too, Mr. Jones," she jokingly said back to him. I was too frightened to laugh. The patient underwent emergency surgery and survived. So did I, but I remember shaking as I drove home that morning.

Sue may have been my charge nurse but she also became a close friend and my mentor. Over the next four years, she gave me so much, both in and out of the hospital. We took classes and studied together. I toasted her marriage and held her firstborn child. When her husband transferred to Germany and we said our last tearful good-byes, I tried to thank her for all she taught me.

"Passing on what I've taught you is the best thanks you can give me," she said. "Be a mentor to a new graduate." I have always remembered those words.

Ten years later, I finally had the opportunity to fulfill Sue's wish when I mentored a new nurse, Dee, in a world-renowned Southern California burn center. Dee also became my friend. When the time came for Dee to move on and she tried to thank me, I remembered Sue and smiled. I told her my story and said the same words to her that Sue said to me.

"Passing on what I've taught you is the best thanks you can give me," I told her. "Be a mentor to a new graduate."

About five years ago, Dee sent me a Christmas card and said she had finally fulfilled the legacy that I had entrusted to her. She had just finished mentoring a new graduate.

This mentoring circle of nursing is closed, yet I know it continues to form new circles as it ripples out to reach other new nurses and other new mentors.

Cecelia Crawford, RN, MSN
Patient Care Services, Pasadena

"The greatest good you can do for another
is not just to share your riches but
to reveal to him his own."
Benjamin Disraeli

Not Just the Diagnosis

My journey began many years ago as an LVN with dreams of becoming an RN. But, as often happens, life got in the way. I married, had children and watched my husband complete his studies. I was finally able to achieve my goal and graduated with my nursing degree in December 2004.

Though I had many years experience, I still came into my new nursing position very much the novice. Expectations of me were now higher. As I started my new career, I first focused on fine-tuning and perfecting the new task-oriented skills I had learned as a student.

As I became more proficient and comfortable in my new role, I started focusing on the psychosocial aspects of nursing care, an area where I'd had very little practice as a student. I felt that I needed to challenge myself in order to meet the needs of my patients better. About eight months into my new career, an opportunity arose that I have never forgotten.

I received my patient assignment and upon getting report was told "good luck with this one." Dread welled up inside of me as I learned that this person had many psychosocial issues along with a terminal medical diagnosis.

"I'm not the right person for this assignment," I thought. "I'm a new graduate. I'm not experienced with the issues facing him." However, I realized that I could not avoid this type of situation forever and decided that I would give it my best shot.

Upon entering the room, the patient barked an order at me to provide him with pain medication. Additionally, I got mistrusting glares from his family. My first instinct was to just get the medication and ignore the rude behavior. Instead, I decided if I was going to develop any kind of relationship with him, that I needed to lay down the ground rules right then.

"I'm more than happy to get your medication but it is not necessary to yell at me," I calmly said. "I am here to help you in any way that I can." He indeed was "difficult" though I preferred to look at him as a person with "high needs."

Caring for him also became a lesson in caring for his family. They were very connected and there was no getting around their involvement. I had to meet their psychosocial needs as well as his. I learned I must consider the family dynamic when caring for a patient.

I went on to develop a trusting relationship with my patient and his family for the remainder of his stay. I learned a great deal from him, primarily to not judge a person. We have no idea what our patients are truly going through unless we have been through it ourselves.

Several months after I had cared for this patient my son received a diagnosis of leukemia. I suddenly became the concerned family member. I was now on the other side of the fence. I would have given anything for my son not to have this serious illness. However, I learned some valuable lessons as I sat by his bedside day after day.

I became acutely aware of the importance of tending to the whole patient and not just the diagnosis. Many times patients are scared and just need someone to talk with them or simply sit quietly by their sides. Sadly, time does not always allow for this important part of care.

Not long after caring for my "high needs" patient, I received a note from his wife thanking me for treating her and her husband with respect and kindness. I had not realized the impact my actions had on them.

Nursing is far more complex than just caring for our patients' physiological needs. We often find ourselves in a position involuntarily attending to the psycho-social needs of both the patient and their family members. We do our patients a great disservice if we don't consider the whole emotional side of their healing as well.

I still consider myself a novice. I hope that I will have many years of nursing ahead of me and there will be many lessons to learn. I am sure the road to becoming an expert will be filled with bumps but I welcome the opportunities to grow and expand my knowledge base. So far, I have found that my life influenced my role as a nurse and being a nurse has influenced my life.

Pamela Reeves, RN
Orange County

*"Always be kind, for everyone is
fighting a hard battle."*
Plato

Reflection

It was September 17, 1999 when I met the Jefferies. As I walked into Richard's hospital room, I noticed his shortness of breath. His wife Dianne looked scared. His doctor just said, "Your pulmonary hypertension symptoms have worsened. The only hope we can give you is Flolan."

"Flo what?" replied Richard.

His doctor said, "Don't worry. You'll learn while you are hospitalized." That is where I came in. I am the nurse educator for Flolan therapy.

A little background first before I continue. As a nurse educator, I teach various intravenous therapies. Some therapies are easy to teach. Then there is Flolan. This delicate drug must be prepared every day by the patient or caregiver. It involves sterile technique to reconstitute it and an intravenous pump to administer it via a special chest catheter. Teaching this therapy is like giving a non-medical person a crash course on being a pharmacist and a nurse.

I assessed if they could commit themselves to this extremely complicated, long-term daily therapy. Richard's manual dexterity was a bit shaky so it was all on Dianne's shoulders. His life was in her hands. Dianne was very scared and nervous, even crying at times as she shared with me her less than perfect life with Richard. This was going to be difficult I thought, but nurses love challenges so I dove right in.

However, this story is not about Richard or Flolan. This is a story about his wife, Dianne. Unbeknownst to both of us, our meeting was to be the start of a long and rewarding journey.

As I worked closely with Dianne, her comfort level gradually increased and her skills kept improving. At the end of the Flolan training, she spoke of an interest in nursing. It is not unusual for a patient or caregiver to get excited about their newly learned skills and when I see that interest, I will encourage them to consider a career in nursing but Dianne surprised me. With so much happening in her personal life, switching careers at that time seemed like it might be more than she could handle.

As the months went by Dianne kept in touch with me. Usually she had questions about Richard's therapy but gradually the conversation turned to questions about becoming a nurse. Then her call came.

"Would you write me a letter of reference?" she said. "I am applying to nursing school." The nurturing relationship that developed between Dianne and me had inspired her.

One day she called my office. "I'm bringing Richard into the clinic today," she said. "Can you meet us afterwards?" We met at a nearby restaurant. When I saw them, they were both beaming.

"I want to show you my nursing school project!" Dianne said.

Out came the most detailed nursing care map I have ever seen. She could hardly contain herself while she explained her work. Meanwhile, Richard sat close to her proudly smiling as she spoke. You had to be there to feel the energy and emotion of that moment. I was so proud of my protégé!

Over the next few years, I monitored her nursing school progress. As her graduation day approached, I received an announcement card. But, it was more than just an invitation to watch her graduate. On June 9, 2005, when they called her name, Richard and I proudly walked up on stage and placed Dianne's nursing school pin on her crisp white uniform.

Her dedication and perseverance inspires me and I would like to think that some of that came about because I inspired her.

Nancy G. Falvo, RN, BSN, CRNI
Department of Education and Training, Los Angeles

"A lot of people have gone further than they thought they could because someone else thought they could."

Unknown

A Tribute to a Mighty Giant

In memory of Raymond M. Kay, MD

A courageous visionary
Kaiser Permanente, a founding father
Despite adversity,
Champion of a new model of care

Pioneer in nurse practitioner education
Committed to collaborative practice
Teams of clinicians,
Together providing care

A gifted listener
Compassionate and trusted by all
Filled with passion and tenacity
Always advocating for what was best

Small in stature
But a giant to all who knew him
My mentor, my colleague
Responsible for my professional journey,
as well as that of many others
The reason many of us are here
reading this book

Linda Fahey, RN, NP, MSN
Regional Manager, Quality and Patient Safety, Patient Care Services, Pasadena

A Love Story

I began, as many of us do, as a medical/surgical ICU nurse. Several years later, I decided to go into maternal/child health nursing, first working in the NICU, then spending 20 years in L&D, and finishing off in the GYN clinic. I met life at its very beginning, welcoming brand-new people into this world.

Now, I am a GYN oncology case manager. Nursing has come full circle for me as I care for women who may be reaching the end of their lives. They may be young, middle-aged or elderly. Each one brings their own special history with them. Often they leave us with very special memories. Such was the case with Ben and Ida.

Ida was a sweet, gentle woman. She and her husband Ben went through two years of surgeries, chemotherapy and radiation. I say it in that manner because Ben never left her side or faltered in any way when it came to her care. He was her hero and her constant tower of strength. Although he was a small man in stature, his love and determination to see his lovely wife cured was all that he needed to keep going. He was a giant in her eyes, as well as in ours.

They never had children and were from a country very far from here. They had only each other, their courageous oncologist and the GYN oncology case manager team.

Ida was having a very difficult time. After so many cycles of chemotherapy, her frail body could barely fight back. She needed to have daily injections of Neupogen to increase her white blood cell count. I had to teach Ben how to give the injections to her.

I arranged to meet with them at their hospital in the outpatient department. When I arrived, they were anxiously awaiting the session. We hugged and chatted, and went into an exam room to begin the lesson. Little did I know it would last for four hours.

Slowly, I reviewed everything about the medication and any possible adverse effects. Ida sat there in her chair, listening and nodding. Ben was the student. He paid careful attention but would always have another question.

Before I knew it, three hours had passed! I handed Ben the make-believe body part, so he could get the "feel" of giving a subcutaneous injection. He pushed the practice tool aside and laughed.

"Why practice? I'll just give it to her now," he said, and he did!

At that moment, the look on Ida's face absolutely sparkled. She beamed from ear to ear, as though Ben had just given her a 10-carat diamond ring! I was so proud of him. He just stood there and smiled, his chest puffed out like a rooster. Ida didn't need to say a word. Her eyes spoke for her. He was her knight in shining armor. He was her hero!

I spent the weekend worrying about whether things went okay. On Monday morning, I phoned Ben. He started laughing uncontrollably. Finally, I asked him what was so funny. He said that his neighbor was a nurse and she offered to give the injections for Ida. He didn't have to give any! I just laughed with him.

A few months later, his beloved Ida died. He was forever at her side, still hoping for a miracle. Her only concern was for Ben's care after she was gone. A few days later, my team partner and I wrote a sympathy card to Ben, expressing how sad we were to have lost Ida.

"I'll always remember her beautiful smile that Friday afternoon when you gave her the injection," I wrote. "She was so proud of you."

A few days later, he called. He was surprised that I had thought so much of that moment. I told him that I would never forget it.

"It was true love at its finest," I said.

He had a tear in his voice when we finally hung up. It had meant a lot to him that I remembered that moment. That instant always hangs in my memory.

Deborah L. Marchica, RN, BSN, PHN
GYN Oncology Case Manager, Bellflower

"To the world, you may just be somebody.
But to somebody, you may just be the world."
Unknown

The Choice

Once upon a time, in a place far, far away, a young lady attended college, studying accounting. Numbers were easy. Her mother was a registered nurse and hoped that someday her daughter would also become a nurse. The young lady refused and refused. Finally, she gave in to her mother's wishes to attend a university nursing school tour. Here the story begins.

The nursing school dorm rooms sure looked good to the young lady. The co-ed students seemed to be happy and having a great time. There were parties planned for each floor. The girl agreed to attend nursing school.

She did not look good in white and the thought of wearing a dress and support hose every day was hard to swallow.

"A nurse's cap!" she thought. "What's that all about?"

Hospitals smelled so medicinal. They were crowded and noisy. There was so much sadness, blood and disease.

"Was nursing really about these things?" she asked herself.

Early days and late hours
Nursing care plans and so much paperwork
Responsibility, oh, so much responsibility

"Life and death situations are nothing like dealing with numbers," she thought and began to doubt her decision.

Then one day, a patient of hers smiled and said, "Thank you" and *got well*. Through her remorse and doubt came this WOW feeling.

"This is great!" she thought. "I have the ability to make a difference."

It was so powerful and so strong. A simple smile made the young woman realize that her choice to be a nurse might be right.

Her nursing school career continued.

Confused patients
Gang members wasting their lives
Leeches needing to be placed in open wounds at 2 a.m.
Maggot-infested surgical sites
Pencil worms floating down rectal tubes
The artificial leg prosthesis being thrown at her
Patients with body lice
Bleeding esophageal varices
The patient presenting with an ax in his skull
Cancer
AIDS
CODE BLUE

"No human being would call this a career. This is more like a horror movie," she thought. Yet, she stayed.

*****

I have now been a registered nurse for almost 26 years. Yet, when it comes right down to it, it is the many stories that I have lived through that have made me stronger, more committed and more compassionate toward my patients.

How could I leave the truck driver who was angry and refused to learn about his newly-diagnosed diabetes only to see him a few months later, having lost weight and in the pharmacy purchasing his diabetic testing supplies? I have made a difference.

What of the elegant woman who traveled the world in search of models for magazines who found out she was dying of metastatic breast cancer; yet, upon admission, she was able to muster up a smile because she was happy to see me!

There were the parents of the young motorcyclist who sustained severe head trauma and kept alive as an organ donor to help so many others. How could I even think of my work as difficult as these parents suffered through the worst fate?

These are just a few experiences from my lengthy career. Many other amazing stories have occurred along my professional path. Each one added to my strength, commitment and compassion.

Nursing is powerful. Having the ability to make a difference and to create positive change is immeasurable. Nursing has the potential to touch so many lives. That young lady, Laura Marcos, long, long ago made the greatest choice ever to become a nurse.

Laura Marcos, RN, BSN
4W, Woodland Hills

"Tell me a fact and I'll learn. Tell me a truth and I'll believe. But tell me a story and it will live in my heart forever."
Indian Proverb

Becoming a Butterfly

I never really wanted to be a nurse. Growing up I wanted to be a veterinarian or a psychologist but as they say, "Life is what happens while you are making other plans."

Approaching 30 and having a brush with cancer made me reevaluate what I wanted in life. Running a payroll department for Los Angeles County was a huge leap from my long lost plans. But quitting my full-time job and going to school for seven years was not in the realm of reality.

Needing a change, I took a career development class that included a battery of tests. I came out very high in medicine. Among the possible choices was professional nurse—two-year program. That course of study seemed like a possibility.

Eventually, I quit my job, paid my bills with my retirement and went off to nursing school. The promised two years became longer because I needed to complete prerequisite course work. But, by carrying 18 units a semester, I was out and working as a nurse in three years.

As I went through school, I felt like a caterpillar that would change into the beautiful butterfly of a nurse. Imagine my dismay when nursing school was over and I didn't feel any different. I passed the boards with double the score I needed but I still didn't feel transformed.

I had determined that I wanted to be a critical care nurse. It looked challenging and stimulating, just the type of work I craved. I was lucky enough to get a critical care internship.

I did well and excelled. Yet upon completion, as I worked in the ICU, if I saw my patient take a turn for the worse, often my first thought was "I better go get the nurse." Then I'd realize, "I am the nurse." I felt like a fraud, not yet having "morphed" into that butterfly.

Then, one day, a young boy was admitted in a coma. He had been drinking at a party. He was 17. He hopped on a motorcycle with his cousin and took off only to hit a tree. His cousin was killed and his life hung in the balance. I would walk by his room and he would be lying there so very still.

One day as I passed by, I noticed that he was tracking me with his eyes. It was so exciting to see there was hope. Soon after, he was moved to my area and I became his nurse.

He was on a ventilator and could not talk, but that didn't stop me. I chatted to him as I worked. It was in the days of one-to-one nursing and I took care of him like a mother cat with one kitten. His mother and his aunt were always there when I came to work.

One night as I began my shift, his mother was not there. I asked his aunt where she was. She told me, "When she saw you come in, she knew he would be all right so she went home." I was so touched by her trust.

I worked with him for days if not weeks. I continuously spoke to him. Never sadly but always full of positive energy. I held his hand as I talked. He had lost a lot of blood and had many transfusions eventually having bleeding problems and never escaping critical condition.

My husband and I took a mini vacation to Santa Barbara. I worried about leaving the boy. That night as I lay in bed miles away, I felt the grasp of that boy's hand in mine. When I awoke the next morning, I called the hospital only to find he had died in the night.

Did he come to say good-bye or was I dreaming? I will never know but I do know it was that boy and many others like him that made me what I am today and what I was really meant to be, a nurse.

Catherine "Cathie" Moore, RN, MHA

Sand Canyon Perioperative Services, Orange County

"Just living is not enough," said the butterfly,
"one must have sunshine, freedom and
a little flower."

Hans Christian Anderson

The Joy and Sadness
of Caring

One evening I was working in our Urgent Appointment Clinic. A middle-aged woman was there with a respiratory complaint and as I listened to her lungs, I noticed a very large, black skin lesion on her right flank.

When I asked her about it, she didn't seem concerned because it had been there, unchanged, for over 15 years. I told her that I was very concerned and insisted that it needed to come off right away! I added her on to my schedule the next day and excised what was the largest skin lesion of its kind that I had ever seen.

The biopsy confirmed what I had feared, malignant melanoma, the most deadly of all skin cancers. I was surprised however to see that, although it was very large, it had not become invasive.

Years later, I was walking down the hall to my office when a woman approached me and asked, "You're PA Sanders aren't you?" I acknowledged that I was and she gave me a big hug. "You saved my life and I was hoping to say thank you in person some day!" she said.

That "thank-you" touched me deeply and continues to remind me of the reasons I chose to practice medicine. It was the greatest reward for caring that one could ever imagine.

* * * * *

A few years ago, a colleague and friend of mine was diagnosed with malignant melanoma. Fortunately, the sentinel nodes were negative, which gave us some hope.

He and I had a number of common interests like old coins and ancient artifacts, and we often consulted with each other on interesting cases. I also worked with both his wife and his daughter in our clinic.

His dry sense of humor was quite evident when you walked into his office and saw a very realistic rubber foot sticking out of a drawer. I chuckled to myself every time I spotted it.

One day he showed me an x-ray of his broken finger. It was obviously a bone tumor, a pathological fracture, in other words a metastasis. My heart sank. He and I both knew this was not a good sign, yet he was very stoic about it.

A few days before Christmas, I went to visit him at his home. At that time, he was considered to be "end-stage" and was rapidly declining. He was in a hospital bed in the living room surrounded by family members. I was at a loss for words.

I sat next to him and put a hand on his forearm. I tried to comfort him by talking about all the lives he had touched and all the people he had helped over the past 40 years.

When I said it must have been hundreds of thousands of patients, he didn't believe me. So I calculated it out for him and then said, "Now do you believe me?" That actually brought a smile to his face and perked him up a bit.

As I left, the night sky was full of magnificent fluffy clouds, brightly backlit by a full moon. I was deeply saddened by the knowledge that my friend would never see another full moon or any of the other simple pleasures of life. I realized that caring and comforting is all one can do at the end of life. That is also why I chose to practice medicine.

Roger J. Sanders, PA
Family Medicine, San Diego

"We cannot direct the wind but we can adjust the sails."
Author Unknown

The Foot Massage

Do you know those days that make you wonder why you became a nurse? Well, for me it was one of those days. I guess it was just my turn. I was hoping to avoid looking after the one anxious patient on the unit but he was mine. So I just took a deep breath and plunged into my much dreaded 12-hour day.

As I walked into my patient's room, I could hear the alarms ringing. I looked at him, trached, with his eyes wide open as I desperately attempted to decipher the words that he was mouthing. After a few moments, it finally came to me like a bolt of lightning, "I can't breathe!" was what he was trying to say.

He appeared to be breathing rapidly but as I glanced at the monitor, I noticed his oxygen saturation was 99% on humidified room air. A quick assessment convinced me he was all right.

"You're fine," I reassured him but it only made matters worse.

"I said I can't breathe!" he mouthed, this time in slow motion with his eyes nearly popping out of his face.

I got on the phone and spoke to his doctor. Soon he too was at the bedside. Realizing that the patient was experiencing an anxiety attack, the doctor ordered some medication that would help my patient relax.

"Ativan, 1 milligram IV push, every four hours as needed for anxiety," he said.

Six hours had passed and my feet were tired. The doctor returned to check on my patient. As he walked into the room, there was a sense of healing in the air. The sun was shining through the window as my patient smiled and nodded his head, acknowledging the doctor's presence. My patient was as calm as a bird. The doctor approached me as I settled my weary feet at the nursing station.

"So, you gave him a dose of ativan?" he asked with a sigh of relief.

"No," I said shaking my head, "I gave him a foot massage."

The doctor looked at me with bewildered eyes, chuckled and walked away smiling. Then I remembered why I became a nurse, because no amount of medication can heal an anxious patient in the way a nurse's heart can.

Maryjo Pulmano, RN, OCN
Charge Nurse, Step Down Unit, Baldwin Park

*"Skilled nurses use their hands, while
good nurses use their minds; but if you
want to be a great nurse, you're going to
have to use your heart."*
Maryjo Pulmano

No One is Indispensable

I have told this story many times because it was one of those unforgettable moments. I changed, and the way I work changed. I have shared it in an effort to help others just as a special colleague and nursing leader helped me.

As the perinatal clinical educator, I was part of the nursing management team that opened Kaiser Permanente Woodland Hills in 1986. During the first few months, I spent most of my time on the OB floors helping nurses learn new systems, equipment and processes. I was feeling a lot of pressure.

One particular afternoon I was sitting in a conference room with an experienced nursing colleague who had served in numerous roles. She was someone I considered a leader and mentor. I told her that I felt as though I had to be on the floors all the time or something would go wrong.

"You know Chris, no one is indispensable," she said with a smile. "If you got appendicitis on the way to work and weren't here tomorrow, the really important things would get done. Perhaps not the way you would have done them, or as well as you would have done them, but things would be okay and people would be okay."

My first thought when I heard this wisdom was that she was right and an enormous weight lifted off my shoulders. It was true, the nurses would figure out the most important things. But her words had another effect as well. I realized that unexpected things can and do happen and one of my jobs was to make sure that what I did could continue whether I was there or not. I needed to put a plan in place so things could go on with or without me.

Since then, as I've begun every job I've ever had, I plan for that unexpected emergency and for my replacement. I train people and put systems in place such that if I suddenly couldn't do my work, others could pick it up and continue it without any adverse effects to Kaiser Permanente or our members.

When I help people learn to do something or provide instructions on how to do something versus doing it for them, it also helps me balance work and life. When I recognize that I am dispensable and I develop ways for others to do what I do, it gives me freedom to enjoy my life. I believe this process makes me a better worker, manager and leader. It has worked well over the years, benefiting both me as well as Kaiser Permanente.

Chris Jones, RN, MBA
Senior Management Consultant, Clinical Decision and
Information Systems, Pasadena

"Do not follow where the path may lead.
Go instead where there is no path and
leave a trail."
Muriel Strode

The Way It's Supposed To Be

I heard the click of the lock and the door opened wide enough for me to see the scrawny, gray-haired man with the coke-bottle thick lenses that magnified his blue eyes, fixing me with a dark glare.

"You were supposed to be here at eleven," Hiram said, stepping aside to let me pass. He gestured towards the formica table in the shared dining area of the house where he rented a room.

I sat down and surveyed the man across from me. He was 75 years old, dressed in blue work clothes, a black belt and shoes from the Army Surplus store. I knew it was the uniform he had worn every day of his adult life. On cold days, he added a blue flight jacket with a fake fur collar.

He was dying of prostate cancer, had metastasis to the bone and lungs and was in major denial. He had never married and hadn't seen any of his brothers or sisters for more than thirty years.

His doctor discharged him from the hospital on the condition that he agreed to hospice so that someone could look after him. He signed on and promptly refused visits from anyone but me, the nurse, on Mondays, Wednesdays and Fridays at eleven in the morning.

"I'm sorry I couldn't get here on time. One of the other people I'm assigned had an emergency," I explained. "I would have called but you don't have a phone."

"I have things to do," he said to me. "I get up at 4:26 a.m. I get dressed, wash my face, then go to the Salt and Pepper to get coffee and read the paper. I come back here at 5:35 a.m. to shave and then I go to Keno's to get my eggs. When I'm done, I come back here and rest until you get here at eleven. That's the way it's supposed to be."

I knew he lived by a set of rigid rules and there was no way I was going to get him to understand, so I opened my bag and got out the necessary items to do an assessment.

"It's just the way it's supposed to be," Hiram continued. "You come at eleven on Monday, Wednesday and Friday. I go to the Little Professor Book Store in Fullerton on the 15th of every month to buy my six magazines. I go to Pull Your Part Auto Salvage Yard on Saturday. On Thursday, I go to the Old Town Buffet with Bob."

I took his vital signs and asked the usual questions. Hiram responded almost before I asked them. He knew the routine. I was soon finished with my assessment.

"Let's talk some more about you taking that plane trip back to Kansas to see your sisters and brother," I said. Hiram bought airplane magazines every month but had never been on a plane in his life.

"I brought you the address of the travel agent I told you about," I said. "She's a nice lady and will help you plan your trip. Are you ready to do it?"

I was floored when he told me he had decided to take me up on my suggestion and fly back to Kansas. I had really hoped he would stay there with his family until he died since he was so alone here in California, but he didn't.

He did, however, have a wonderful time and didn't stop talking about the airplane ride until he died. It was so gratifying to me to know that I was able to make a difference in his last few months of life and not necessarily in the usual way that nurses make a difference.

Kathy Pratt, RN, BSN, PHN
Hospice, Bellflower

"Too often we underestimate the power of a touch, a smile, a kind word, a listening ear, an honest compliment, or the smallest act of caring, all of which have the potential to turn a life around."

Leo F. Buscaglia

Surrounded by Angels

On an ordinary workday, I am in my scrubs, fully equipped with my stethoscope and a few alcohol swabs stuffed in my pockets. I am ready for the next emergency, a drop in blood pressure or a change in level of consciousness. I always believed that I was prepared until the day the patient I was watching was my own son.

The very day he was born, I knew he would have to have surgery to repair the hole in his heart. His doctors warned me he would need the operation when he turned one. Now, one year's time had passed, but I was not ready.

The day came and a woman with long blonde hair and sky blue scrubs approached my husband and me.

"I'm going to be your son's anesthesiologist," she said with a sweet smile. "I'm going to give him some medication that will make him sleepy."

As we took one last look at him, I slowly shifted him from my arms into hers. I watched her walk away holding my son, vanishing into the white walls of the hospital corridor. I turned to my husband with empty arms and tears rolling down my face. Seconds had passed, then minutes, then hours. There was not much we could do except hold each other and pray.

Just when my eyes grew weary, a messenger came to visit. "He is going to be alright," she said. As she turned the other way, I heard a sound that seemed to come closer. A group of three people, dressed in scrubs, diligently pushed the bed on which my son was peacefully resting. I could hear the promising sound of his heart monitor drifting past me. As they settled him into his room, my husband and I watched the rising and falling of his chest.

"A sign of life," I whispered as I moved to his bedside. I fell asleep watching him breathe.

Another lady dressed in bright red scrubs patiently arranged all the tubes that were attached to him. She smiled at me as I watched her take over his care. This time I was merely a spectator. Finding myself enclosed within the white walls of an unfamiliar hospital, I watched many people in scrubs take turns caring for my son. A straight-haired woman made puppets out of tongue blades and a rattle out of a specimen cup. When I saw my son's eyes brighten up, I knew he was alright. When I heard him giggle, it was as though a promise had been fulfilled.

Two mornings after his surgery, another lady in pink scrubs approached me holding him at her waist.

"He wouldn't let me put him down so I just carried him around," she said laughing light-heartedly. "Oh, and the doctor said he can go home today," she continued.

Her last words rang in my ears like the sound of school bells on the first day of summer break. She stretched her arms out and gently laid him into my yearning embrace.

As my husband and I drove home with our son later that day, I began to ponder. I was humbled and convinced that my son had been surrounded by angels dressed in scrubs.

Maryjo Pulmano, RN, OCN
Charge Nurse, Step Down Unit, Baldwin Park

"A kind heart is a fountain of gladness,
making everything in its vicinity into smiles."
Washington Irving

Life is So Short

In June 2007, my husband was diagnosed with lymphoma. We found out from a lymph node biopsy. His illness was unexpected. His treatment consisted of six doses of chemotherapy. He had a bone marrow test and his chemotherapy started in July. We anticipated recovery.

He tolerated the first and second chemotherapy doses well. After the third treatment, however, he started getting sick. He lost twenty pounds, his white count was very low, his temperature was constantly very high and acetaminophen did not help. Then he was admitted into the hospital with sepsis, which was possibly due to a port-a-cath infection. He had antibiotic treatment and stayed in the hospital for three days.

After his discharge, I had to take total care of him at home. Along with antibiotics, tube feeding and insulin to control his blood sugar, he needed a bedside commode and a walker. I tried to help him get his strength back but he was very weak.

After the fourth chemotherapy dose, he was admitted to ICU because his blood sugar dropped below 30 and he was semiconscious. After one week, he came home with more antibiotics. By August, I had taken family leave from work to provide 24-hour care.

He became even sicker with the fifth and sixth chemotherapy treatments. He had nausea and vomiting. He could not even keep fluids down. I also noticed that he looked yellow and jaundiced.

I took him to the emergency room soon after Christmas. They gave him TPN and lipid treatment. He was unable to help himself at this time and was under total care. He was using diapers around the clock. My family and I spent New Years in the hospital. His condition continued to get worse.

On the night of January 4, he had a cardiac arrest. Early the next morning of January 5, he died at the age of 62. I let him take his last breaths because he did not wish to have intubation. My sister, my son, my daughter and I were there at his bedside until he passed away.

It has now been almost a year since his death. I have had some time to process what happened and gain a bit of perspective. I realized that my knowledge and experience as a nurse enabled me to help him, spend time with him and make him feel more comfortable throughout his terrible illness until the last minutes of his life.

My skill and ability allowed me to know and understand the situation. I was able to prepare myself and my family for what was coming. Caring for my husband made me appreciate life more because unexpected things like his illness can happen so suddenly. I have gathered resilience and strength, and have surrounded my children with caring and love as we begin to move toward our future.

Kanlaya Wongthipkongka, RN
Manager, Nursing Administration, Fontana

"Love is more than a noun—it is a verb;
it is more than a feeling—it is caring,
sharing, helping, sacrificing."
William Arthur Ward

The Boy Named Sue

As an OB/GYN nurse practitioner, I encountered many patients with a variety of medical problems and issues, but my favorites were always the moms pregnant for the first time.

My last patient of the day was a young woman who I had seen through most of her pregnancy. She was 32-weeks along, expecting her first child (a boy) and loved being pregnant. Frequently her husband would come with her and at each visit she was bubbling over with questions.

As I walked into the examination room, I noticed she was alone this time and very quiet without her usual smile. I asked her the routine questions and she responded. I did her exam and the baby was fine. Then I sat down.

"What's wrong?" I asked.

"Nothing," she said but I noticed she could not look me in the eye.

"I think something is bothering you," I persisted.

"It's nothing," she answered again.

"Okay," I said. "I can tell something is wrong. Let's talk about it. I care about you."

And with that, her tears started. She told me she was physically abused by her husband and afraid to tell anyone. She said that he was threatening her and controlled where she went and who she saw. Coming to Kaiser Permanente and seeing me was the highlight of her life.

"It doesn't matter about me," she said. "I am afraid that he will hurt the baby."

I knew that the hardest part of the conversation was yet to come. Did she want us to help her get away from him and move to a safe place? I knew that frequently abused women are not ready to leave and are very frightened of the abuser. I knew because I had been there too.

It was my secret and only a few people knew about it. But, in that moment, I knew I needed to share what happened to me. I told her my story of survival and that there would be light at the end of the tunnel of despair.

With her permission, we consulted with the social worker and found her a safe haven. I helped her call her sister to start the communication with her family and to let out the secret she had held for so long so it could no longer have the power to control her life.

We kept in touch over the following weeks, with many tears and long conversations. After so many years, it amazed me how my emotions came flooding back but I was determined to be the support she needed to be a survivor too.

As a part of her recovery, she moved out of town. I soon received a card announcing the birth of her long-awaited baby boy who she jokingly said would always be known in her heart as the boy named Sue.

Sue Al-Sabih, NP, MSN
Practice Leader, SCPMG Ambulatory Clinical Services, Pasadena

"Love and compassion are necessities, not luxuries.
Without them humanity cannot survive."
Dalai Lama

The Great Teacher

I had returned to graduate school and, being of the "if-I-am-going-to-do-something-I-am-going-do-it-in-the-shortest-possible-time" nature, I was carrying a full load of 12 units. At the time, I was newly married and recently promoted to a coordinator position of a small hospice team. In addition to working four 10-hour days per week, I was also on-call for a week at a time every other week. I managed to keep this routine up for about a year, until things came to a head one fall evening.

I had a class from 6 p.m. to 10 p.m. at California State University, Los Angeles. I parked in my usual parking area at the bottom of Cardiac Hill, informally named by students because the climb to the campus from the parking lot was 10 flights of stairs. I had just gotten to my class, when I received a page and responded to a call from the grandson of one of our hospice patients.

As the young man described the situation, I was sure his grandmother was nearing the end of her life. Though I had not met her, the hospice team had anticipated this event so as the nurse-on-call, I was not surprised. I asked if he would like me to visit. He declined, indicating that there were many family members present and they were taking turns sitting with his grandmother. I asked him to call me if anything changed.

About an hour after my class started, I received another page. It was a call from the same patient's home. I responded and spoke to the grandson again. He told me that his grandmother was quiet now, her respirations had stopped and he thought she had died. I told him I would be there to assist them. It was at that moment that I fell apart and began to feel sorry for myself.

As I walked across campus and back down Cardiac Hill, I started to weep. In my mind, I played and re-played, over and over, how tired I was and my annoyance that I had to leave my class. "Why did she have to die now?" rolled around in my brain incessantly.

By the time I got into my car, I was crying uncontrollably. All the stress of work, school and very little free time caught up with me. I sobbed all the way down the Long Beach freeway to Paramount, where this patient had lived.

As I drove up to the house, I remember thinking, "I can't let this family know I was crying." I wiped my eyes, blew my nose, patted my cheeks and began to pull myself together. As I got out of the car, I noticed the many extended family members sitting outside the house and spilling out the door. I walked up to the house and the grandson greeted me.

He thanked me for coming and I went in to see his grandmother. As I went through the process of pronouncing the death of the family matriarch, the honor of being in that place, at that time struck me. Suddenly, my own fatigue and anxiety paled in the presence of the love this extended family had for their mother, grandmother, aunt and friend. I was humbled to assist them in final preparations, and more humbled as I heard this one unique and special family reviewing her life.

I spent a brief hour and a half with that family before the representatives from the mortuary came. In that short time, I learned much about the value of human interactions and relationships, and about prioritizing what is important in this life. Twenty years later I still hold in my heart the lessons I learned that night. Names fade, but feelings are forever.

Kris Hillary, NP, MSN
Regional Director, Home Care Services, Pasadena

"We must be willing to let go of the life we planned
so as to have the life that is waiting for us."
E.M. Forster

Postmortem

I guess I was fortunate to be in an ADN program that taught postmortem care as a skills lab module, as well as part of our first year clinical performance. I remember the first time I participated in the postmortem care of a patient in my second semester of clinical. My instructor gathered three students and we quietly entered the patient's room. We bathed the patient, positioned him and shrouded him per hospital policy. But what I remember most was the reverence the instructor insisted upon during these tasks.

"This is the last act of nursing care you will give to this patient," she said to us. "Do it with dignity and honor the person who once existed just a few moments ago."

I had a chance to remember those words as a new graduate. I was the night shift charge nurse of a 40-bed surgical floor, one of two RNs with three LVNs rounding out the team. (How on earth did we ever do that?) As a new graduate, of course I was a concrete thinker focused on task completion and was very goal directed.

An elderly woman, the matriarch of her family, died at the beginning of the shift with her family members at the bedside. The family originated from the Appalachia Mountains and had a family tradition of bathing the newly deceased person before burial. Not just one bath—each person bathed the deceased, one at a time. Even children participated in this ritual.

When I was informed that the family would be performing this lengthy procedure, all I could think of was "How am I going to get the body to the morgue in the two hours dictated by policy?" However, soon I found myself fascinated by the family postmortem care. In-between my other patient care responsibilities, I kept coming back to the room to silently watch each family member express their love to the matriarch as they each bathed her.

The last person to bathe the deceased patient was the 6-year-old great-granddaughter. I was very concerned at the beginning of this ritual about a young child's ability to handle this emotionally exhausting experience. However, the role modeling demonstrated by the brothers, sisters, children and grandchildren prepared the child and allowed her to participate in this important family function. She was asked only to wash the face and hands of her Granny. Tears welled in my eyes as I heard her whisper, "I love you Granny. I'll miss you."

When she finished, the entire family praised her, but she was looking to her mother for a final confirmation of her actions. "Mommy, did I do good?" she asked. Her mother hugged her and said, "You did so good, honey. Now Granny is clean and can go to God." The child just beamed. She was truly part of her family now. I remembered the words of my clinical instructor and never again rushed a family from their last moments with their deceased loved one.

I doubt bathing the deceased is even part of current postmortem care. This is the ONLY time I have witnessed a family give any part of postmortem care. I have always wondered if families would participate in this last and final act of hospitalization. Maybe not—the modern disconnect from the act of death may make this a moot point. This event made such an impact on my professional nursing career that I felt I must share it.

Cecelia Crawford, RN, MSN

Patient Care Services, Pasadena

"The real depths of nursing can only be made known
through ideals, love, sympathy, knowledge, and culture,
and expressed through the practice of
artistic procedures and relationships."

Euphemia Jane Taylor

Wedding Cake for Olga

Olga was my first patient as an RN, a "Real Nurse." I had just graduated and was working in a skilled nursing facility. I love geriatrics. I worked the evening shift and my soon-to-be husband Neil would come and bring me dinner. Olga, a long-time resident, would always come into the lounge and have coffee with us as we ate. She soon became my favorite patient because of her blue eyes, warm smile and great stories about when she was "young and wild" as Olga would say.

My husband-to-be and I were making wedding plans one evening on a quick dinner break. The cake was the topic of discussion. "What kind of cake would you like?" my fiancé asked me.

Before I could even answer, Olga quickly replied, "Carrot cake, sweetie!"

We all started laughing. We had decided to invite Olga and her family to the wedding as our special guests. Olga was very excited but when our wedding day came, Olga was too frail to go. Both my fiancé and I were disappointed that she could not attend since she had been so involved in the conversations around the planning of the big event.

Our wedding was beautiful but it was ending. The guests had departed with fond farewells, hugs and kisses, and well wishes for a happy future when we decided to deliver some wedding cake to Olga.

She was thrilled. Her blue eyes beamed and her warm smile greeted us when we walked into the nursing station with food, favors and cake. We sat and chatted with her about the wedding while she ate her slice of wedding cake, and yes—it was carrot cake!

We took some time from a day that meant the world to us and gave her a moment that meant the world to her. She greeted me with a chorus of "Here Comes the Bride" and her warm blue-eyed smile on my first day back to work after returning from my honeymoon. I will never forget Olga. I remember her every time I eat carrot cake.

Susan Mattera, RN, MN
Area Administrator, Home Care, Los Angeles

*"Depth of friendship does not depend on
length of acquaintance."*
Rabindranath Tagore

Definitely an Angel

From a patient letter

On April 17, 2007, we found out that our son RJ had a brain tumor. He had surgery to remove it but the pathology report revealed that it was malignant. After speaking with his doctor, we decided that he would undergo chemotherapy, which meant spending the next seven months in the hospital. The very thought seemed like an eternity and we wondered how we would make it through.

It was the wonderful nursing staff at Kaiser Permanente Los Angeles that came to our rescue and helped make the days go by easily. One nurse, Virgie Navarette, made it a point to visit RJ daily. She would come into his room with her great smile and ask, "How's my man doing?" She would often sit down to share a meal and play games with him.

Every morning when RJ woke up, he would stare out of his window looking at the Griffith Park Observatory. He would tell me daily, "Mom I want to go there," and my response was, "RJ, when you get better, we will all go."

As I was talking to him, Virgie was making her daily visit to RJ. She asked him what was wrong. He pointed and told her that he wanted to go to that big, white house when he was feeling better. "I don't think it's fair that you have to wait," she said. "Let me see what I can do." She wanted to make him happy right then.

With a few phone calls, Virgie made his dream come true. She contacted the council member for that district, who was a friend of hers and told him about the situation. Between the two of them, they made an extraordinary outing possible.

October 24, 2007 was the chosen day. We pulled in front of the hospital to pick up RJ. Greeting us along with Virgie and other nursing staff were the council member and firefighters with their very large, very red-hook-and-ladder truck. RJ was standing there speechless but he had the biggest smile you have ever seen. He received royal treatment. RJ rode in the fire truck to the observatory and our family had a special tour.

Virgie is definitely an angel. She granted a wish and put a smile on RJ's face. I know that my child has a special place in her heart. I thank her immensely for loving my RJ and making him the happiest little boy in town. God definitely knew what he was doing when he made her a nurse because she is nurturing, kind spirited and big hearted. Thank you, thank you.

With Warmest Regards,
Tanya Watson

Virgie is the Clinical Nurse Coordinator for Pediatrics/PICU at Kaiser Permanente Los Angeles. She has been with Kaiser Permanente 29 years. She was a DAISY Award recipient in 2008.

Submitted by:
Mindy C. Ofiana, RN, MSN
Director, Critical Care Services, Los Angeles

*"Where there is great love
there are always miracles."*

Willa Cather

The Gift of a New Year

I was working in an NICU at a major medical center. During one Thanksgiving week, a family from Canada transferred to our facility to deliver their conjoined twin girls. They were born by cesarean section a day or two before the holiday. Their connection was at the chest, one of the most difficult places for conjoined twins. It was quickly determined that they shared a heart, liver and intestines. They faced each other. It was cute to see them playing and looking at each other. They were both intubated and on a ventilator.

The parents and "big sister" (all of about 3 years old) joined our unit for Thanksgiving dinner since they were from out of town and living in a motel. The family stayed in the area for a few weeks. However, it became obvious that eventually the parents and sister would have to return home. They decided that the mother and daughter would go back and the father would stay. They left after Christmas leaving the father to be close to the babies.

As the New Year approached, I found myself with two tickets to the Rose Bowl game between the University of Southern California and the University of Michigan. I had gotten close to the family because I was the primary nurse caring for the babies. One day, as I was caring for them and the father was at the bedside, I asked him if he liked football. I wasn't sure if Canada was a big football country like the United States. He said "yes." I told him that I had two tickets to the game and asked him if he would like to go.

One of the neonatologists overheard our conversation and said that he lived in Pasadena, within walking distance of the parade. If we wanted, he said we could join his family for breakfast, walk to the parade, and he would drive us to and from the game. This sounded like fun.

So on New Year's morning, I picked up the father at his motel. We drove to the physician's home, had breakfast with his family, went to the parade and then to the game. Our seats were on the end zone so we could root for both teams. After the game, we returned to the physician's house for dinner. It was a great way to start a new year. The father later thanked us for the wonderful day. It allowed him to get out of the NICU for a little fun and away from his stress for a few hours.

Since that day, the New Year's Rose Parade and Bowl Game have always had a special meaning to me and hold a memorable place in my heart. I will always remember the family. Unfortunately, the babies were unable to be parted successfully and they both died during the separation surgery a few months later. However, as a nurse, I know that for the short time they were with us, they were loved by their parents and especially by the staff (including me) of the NICU.

Randy Retin Miller, RN, BS
Manager, Staff Education, Panorama City

"*Fashion your life as a garland of
beautiful deeds.*"
Buddha

The Value of Nursing

I touch the lives of young and old
I make a difference so I'm told
I provide support and educate
For the patient, I advocate

I manage skills of complexity
In a myriad of role diversity
I perform at levels which you cannot rehearse
I respect my value, I am a nurse

Inez Tenzer, RN, PhD (1943–2007)
Written in honor of Nurse Recognition Week, May 1993

Books on Storytelling and Other Matters

Armstrong, David M.
Managing by Storying Around:
A New Method of Leadership

Blanchard, Ken and Barbara Glanz
The Simple Truths of Service

DePree, Max
Leadership Is An Art

DePree, Max
Leading Without Power

Hammerschlag, Carl A., MD
The Dancing Healers

Koerner, JoEllen
Healing Presence: The Essence of Nursing

Koerner, JoEllen
Mother, Heal My Self: An Intergenerational
Healing Journey Between Two Worlds

Kouzes, James M. and Barry Z. Posner
Encouraging the Heart

Lee, Fred
If Disney Ran Your Hospital:
9½ Things You Would Do Differently

Lipman, Doug
The Storytelling Coach: How to Listen, Praise,
and Bring Out People's Best

Maguire, Jack
The Power of Personal Storytelling

Neuhauser, Peg C.
Corporate Legends and Lore: The Power of
Storytelling as a Management Tool

Remen, Rachel Naomi
Kitchen Table Wisdom: Stories That Heal

Selzer, Richard
Letters to a Young Doctor

Simmons, Annette
The Story Factor

Stone, Richard D.
The Healing Art of Storytelling:
A Sacred Journey of Personal Discovery

Studer, Quint
What's Right in Health Care: 365 Stories of
Purpose, Worthwhile Work, and Making
a Difference

**Styles, Margretta Madden and Patricia
Moccia**
On Nursing: A Literary Celebration

**Zander, Rosamund Stone and
Benjamin Zander**
The Art of Possibility: Transforming
Professional and Personal Life

Guide to Abbreviations

A1C—Hemoglobin A1C, a blood test that shows a three-month average blood sugar in patients with diabetes

ADA—Assistant Department Administrator

ADN—Associate Degree in Nursing

AIDS—Acquired Immune Deficiency Syndrome

ALS—Amyotrophic Lateral Sclerosis, Lou Gehrig's disease

BMI—Body Mass Index

BSN—Bachelor of Science in Nursing

C-Section—Cesarean Section

CAT Scan—Computed Axial Tomography

CCRN—Certification for Adult, Neonatal and Pediatric Critical Care Nurses

CCU—Cardiac Care Unit

CHP—California Highway Patrol

CNA—Certified Nursing Assistant

CNM—Certified Nurse-Midwife

CNS—Clinical Nurse Specialist

Code Blue—A call for medical personnel and equipment to resuscitate a patient

CNOR—Certified Nurse Operating Room

COPD—Chronic Obstructive Pulmonary Disease

CPR—Cardiopulmonary Resuscitation

CPSN—Certified Plastic Surgical Nurse

CRNA—Certified Registered Nurse Anesthetist

CRNI—Certified Registered Nurse Infusion

C-Spine—Cervical Spine

CT—Computed Tomography

DA—Department Administrator

DAISY—Diseases Attacking the Immune System, the DAISY Award recognizes extraordinary nurses

DO—Doctor of Osteopathic Medicine

ED—Emergency Department

ER—Emergency Room

FNP—Family Nurse Practitioner

GI—Gastrointestinal

GYN—Gynecology

HIV—Human Immunodeficiency Virus

ICU—Intensive Care Unit

INR Results—International Normalized Ratio, a test to monitor how long it takes blood to clot

IV—Intravenous

L&D—Labor and Delivery

LCSW—Licensed Clinical Social Worker

LSAT—Law School Admission Test

LVN—Licensed Vocational Nurse

MA—Master of Arts

M.Div.—Master of Divinity

MBA—Master of Business Administration

mg—Milligram

MHA—Master of Health Administration

MI—Myocardial Infarction (heart attack)

ml—Milliliter

MN—Master of Nursing

MPA—Master of Public Administration

MPH—Master of Public Health

MRI—Magnetic Resonance Imaging

MSN—Master of Science, Nursing

MSPAS—Master of Science, Physician Assistant Studies

MSW—Master of Social Work

NICU—Neonatal Intensive Care Unit

NP—Nurse Practitioner

OB—Obstetrics

OB/GYN—Obstetrics/Gynecology

OCN— Oncology Certified Nurse

OR—Operating Room

PA—Physician Assistant

PA-C—Physician Assistant—Certified

Pap—Papanicolaou Test for Cervical Cancer

PhD—Doctor of Philosophy

PHN—Public Health Nurse

PICC Line—Peripherally Inserted Central Catheter

PICU—Pediatric Intensive Care Unit

RN—Registered Nurse

RN-BC—Registered Nurse—Board Certified

RNC—Registered Nurse, Certified

SCPMG—Southern California Permanente Medical Group

SDA—Same Day Admit

SNF—Skilled Nursing Facility

SRNA—Student Registered Nurse Anesthetist

STAT—Medical term for "immediate"

TPN—Total Parenteral Nutrition

Quotes by Subject

Beginnings

How wonderful it is that nobody need wait a single moment before starting to improve the world. *Anne Frank*

I never lose an opportunity of urging a practical beginning, however small, for it is wonderful how often the mustard seed germinates and roots itself.
Florence Nightingale

Caring

Caring about others, running the risk of feeling, and leaving an impact on people, brings happiness. *Harold Kushner*

Caring is a reflex. Someone slips, your arm goes out. A car is in the ditch, you join the others and push...You live, you help. *Ram Dass*

Caring is the shining thread of gold that holds together the tapestry of life.
Ida V. Moffett

Cure sometimes, treat often, comfort always.
Hippocrates

I feel the capacity to care is the thing which gives life its deepest significance.
Pablo Casals

In compassion lies the world's true strength. *Buddha*

It is a beautiful and mysterious power that one human being can have on another through the mere act of caring....A great truth, the act of caring is the first step in the power to heal. *Phillip Moffitt*

"Just living is not enough," said the butterfly, "one must have sunshine, freedom and a little flower." *Hans Christian Anderson*

Too often we underestimate the power of a touch, a smile, a kind word, a listening ear, an honest compliment, or the smallest act of caring, all of which have the potential to turn a life around. *Leo F. Buscaglia*

Unless someone like you cares a whole awful lot, nothing is going to get better. It's not. *Dr. Seuss*

Cats

I love cats because I love my home and after awhile they become its visible soul. *Jean Cocteau*

No amount of time can erase the memory of a good cat, and no amount of masking tape can ever totally remove his fur from your couch. *Leo Dworken*

Children

A child is a gift whose worth cannot be measured except by the heart. *Theresa Ann Hunt*

While we try to teach our children all about life, our children teach us what life is all about. *Unknown*

Commitment

There's a difference between interest and commitment. When you're interested in doing something, you do it only when it's convenient. When you're committed to something, you accept no excuses; only results. *Kenneth Blanchard*

Death

Death ends a life, not a relationship. *Robert Benchley*

Death leaves a heartache no one can heal, love leaves a memory no one can steal. *From a headstone in Ireland*

Deeds

Fashion your life as a garland of beautiful deeds. *Buddha*

How far that little candle throws his beams! So shines a good deed in a weary world. *William Shakespeare*

One of the things I keep learning is that the secret of being happy is doing things for other people. *Dick Gregory*

Since you cannot do good to all, you are to pay special attention to those who, by the accidents of time, or place, or circumstances, are brought into closer connection with you. *Augustine of Hippo*

There are two ways of spreading light: to be the candle or the mirror that reflects it. *Edith Wharton*

Dreams

Go confidently in the direction of your dreams. Live the life you've imagined. *Henry David Thoreau*

Faith

More things are wrought by prayer than this world dreams of. *Alfred, Lord Tennyson*

Without faith, nothing is possible. With it, nothing is impossible. *Mary Mcleod Bethune*

Friendship

Depth of friendship does not depend on length of acquaintance. *Rabindranath Tagore*

I am a part of all that I have met. *Alfred, Lord Tennyson*

Remember that everyone you meet is afraid of something, loves something and has lost something. *H. Jackson Brown, Jr.*

Giving

A bit of fragrance always clings to the hand that gives roses. *Chinese Proverb*

Happiness

Happiness cannot come from without. It must come from within. It is not what we see and touch or that which others do for us which makes us happy; it is that which we think and feel and do, first for the other fellow and then for ourselves. *Helen Keller*

Heart

The best and most beautiful things in life cannot be seen, not touched, but are felt in the heart. *Helen Keller*

Humor

Humor is the great thing, the saving thing. The minute it crops up, all our irritations and resentments slip away and a sunny spirit takes their place. *Mark Twain*

Kindness

A kind heart is a fountain of gladness, making everything in its vicinity into smiles. *Washington Irving*

Always be kind, for everyone is fighting a hard battle. *Plato*

If you have not often felt the joy of doing a kind act, you have neglected much, and most of all yourself. *A. Neilen*

Kind words can be short and easy to speak, but their echoes are truly endless. *Mother Teresa*

Kind words do not cost much. Yet they accomplish much. *Blaise Pascal*

Kindness in words creates confidence. Kindness in thinking creates profoundness. Kindness in giving creates love. *Lao Tzu*

Kindness is the golden chain by which society is bound together. *Goethe*

No act of kindness, however small, is ever wasted. *Aesop*

Remember there's no such thing as a small act of kindness. Every act creates a ripple with no logical end. *Scott Adams*

This is my simple religion. There is no need for temples; no need for complicated philosophy. Our own brain, our own heart is our temple; the philosophy is kindness. *Dalai Lama*

Wherever there is a human being, there is an opportunity for a kindness. *Seneca*

Life

Because I have loved life, I shall have no sorrow to die. *Amelia Burr*

The only thing that should surprise us is that there are still some things that can surprise us. *Francois De La Rochefoucauld*

The true meaning of life is to plant trees under whose shade you do not expect to sit. *Nelson Henderson*

To each age comes its own peculiar problems and challenges, but to it also comes the necessary vision and strength. *Ruth Weaver Hubbard*

When we share—that is poetry in the prose of life. *Sigmund Freud*

Love

Love and compassion are necessities, not luxuries. Without them humanity cannot survive. *Dalai Lama*

Love is more than a noun—it is a verb; it is more than a feeling—it is caring, sharing, helping, sacrificing. *William Arthur Ward*

To the world, you may just be somebody. But to somebody, you may just be the world. *Unknown*

We can do no great things, only small things with great love. *Mother Teresa*

Where there is great love there are always miracles. *Willa Cather*

We need four hugs a day for survival. We need eight hugs a day for maintenance. We need twelve hugs a day for growth. *Virginia Satir*

Making a Difference

People will forget what you said, people will forget what you did, but people will never forget how you made them feel. *Maya Angelou*

We have a choice to use the gift of our life to make the world a better place or not to bother. *Jane Goodall*

We must not, in trying to think about how we can make a big difference, ignore the small daily differences we can make which, over time, add up to big differences that we often cannot foresee. *Marian Wright Edelman*

What we have done for ourselves alone dies with us. What we have done for others and the world remains and is immortal. *Albert Pine*

What you leave behind is not what is engraved in stone monuments, but what is woven into the lives of others. *Pericles*

Mentorship

A lot of people have gone further than they thought they could because someone else thought they could. *Unknown*

Few things in the world are more powerful than a positive push. A smile. A word of optimism and hope. A 'you can do it' when things are tough.
Richard M. De Vos

The greatest good you can do for another is not just to share your riches but to reveal to him his own. *Benjamin Disraeli*

Miracles

I think miracles exist in part as gifts and in part as clues that there is something beyond the flat world we see. *Peggy Noonan*

Miracles come in moments. Be ready and willing. *Wayne Dyer*

There are only two ways to live your life. One is as though nothing is a miracle. The other is as though everything is a miracle. *Albert Einstein*

We are miracles. Each of us is an absolute astonishment. So whether you believe in miracles or not, we still are. We still partake of 'miracledom.' *Ruby Doe*

When we do the best we can, we never know what miracle is wrought in our life, or in the life of another. *Helen Keller*

Mothers and Babies

A mother is a person who seeing there are only four pieces of pie for five people, promptly announces she never did care for pie. *Tenneva Jordan*

A new baby is like the beginning of all things—wonder, hope, a dream of possibilities. *Eda J. Le Shan*

Nurses/Nursing

Nurses are angels in comfortable shoes. *Author Unknown*

Nursing encompasses an art, a humanistic orientation, a feeling for the value of the individual, and an intuitive sense of ethics, and of the appropriateness of action taken. *Myrtle Aydelotte*

Skilled nurses use their hands, while good nurses use their minds; but if you want to be a great nurse, you're going to have to use your heart. *Maryjo Pulmano*

The central concerns of nursing—care, comfort, guidance, and helping individuals cope with health problems—have not changed. *Eleanor Lambertsen*

The real depths of nursing can only be made known through ideals, love, sympathy, knowledge, and culture, and expressed through the practice of artistic procedures and relationships." *Euphemia Jane Taylor*

To do what nobody else will do, in a way that nobody else can do, in spite of all we go through; is to be a nurse. *Rawsi Williams*

Obstacles

Thorns and stings
And those such things
Just make stronger
Our angel wings.
Emme Woodhull-Bäche

We cannot direct the wind but we can adjust the sails. *Author Unknown*

We could never learn to be brave and patient if there were only joy in the world. *Helen Keller*

We must be willing to let go of the life we planned so as to have the life that is waiting for us. *E.M. Forster*

Perseverance

Be like a postage stamp. Stick to something until you get there. *Josh Billings*

Road Less Traveled

Chance is always powerful. Let your hook be always cast; in the pool where you least expect it, there will be a fish. *Ovid*

Do not follow where the path may lead. Go instead where there is no path and leave a trail. *Muriel Strode*

I am only one; but still I am one. I cannot do everything, but still I can do something. I will not refuse to do something I can do. *Helen Keller*

There are no traffic jams when you go the extra mile. *Attributed to both Zig Ziglar and Dr. Kenneth McFarland*

Stories and Song

It takes a thousand voices to tell a single story. *Native American Saying*

Our stories matter…Your stories matter…For you never know how much of a difference they make and to whom. *Caroline Joy Adams*

Our sweetest songs are those that tell of saddest thought. *Percy Bysshe Shelley*

Storytelling is the most powerful way to put ideas into the world today. *Robert McKee*

Tell me a fact and I'll learn. Tell me a truth and I'll believe. But tell me a story and it will live in my heart forever. *Indian proverb*

Thinking/Intuition/Creativity

Anyone can look for fashion in a boutique or history in a museum. The creative explorer looks for history in a hardware store and fashion in an airport. *Robert Wieder*

Intuition is a spiritual faculty and does not explain, but simply points the way. *Florence Scovel Shinn*

Wisdom

Knowledge is learning something every day. Wisdom is letting go of something every day. *Zen Proverb*

We are made wise not by the recollection of our past, but by the responsibility for our future. *George Bernard Shaw*

What is history? An echo of the past in the future; a reflex from the future on the past. *Victor Hugo*

Work

Satisfaction in your work is one of the fruits of a wise choice. *Eugenia Kennedy Spalding*

Index